VAPOR

THE ART AND SCIENCE OF INHALING PURE PLANT ESSENCES

VAPOR

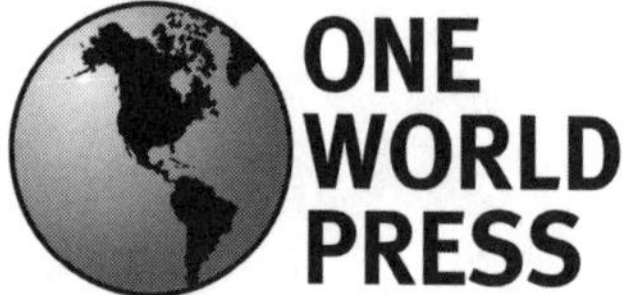

THE ART AND SCIENCE OF INHALING PURE PLANT ESSENCES

SHAAHIN SEAN CHEYENE

Advanced Inhalation Revolutions, Inc.
1041 Pleasantview, Venice, CA 90291
310-581-1312
vapor@air-2.com
www.vapir.com

Cover, layout and design: Hidden Fortress Design Studios
paul@hiddenfortress.net
Library of Congress Cataloging-in-Publication Data
Cheyene, Shaahin Sean, 1975-
Vapor : the science of inhaling plant essences / Shaahin Sean Cheyene.-- 1st ed.
p. ; cm.
Includes bibliographical references and index.
ISBN 0-9644958-8-0 (alk. paper)
1. Aromatherapy. 2. Vapors.
[DNLM: 1. Plant Oils --therapeutic use. 2. Volatilization. 3. Administration, Inhalation. 4. Aromatherapy--methods. WB 925 C531v 2003] I. Title.
RM666.A68 C48 2003
615'.321--dc21

2003006298

ONE WORLD PRESS
1042 Willow Creek Rd., Suite A101-195
Prescott, AZ 86301
800-250-8171
oneworldpress@mail.com

This book was printed in the U.S.A. on recycled paper using soy ink.

03 04 05 06 07 5 4 3 2 1

To Asa

"There is one thing stronger than all the armies in the world,
and that is an idea whose time has come."
Victor Hugo, 1802–1885

Forward

Vapor: The Art & Science of Inhaling Plant Essences introduces one of the most exciting technologies to emerge this century. Digital Vaporization holds the key to increased physical and mental health and well being for millions. This technology (DVT) offers a pure, concentrated method of fortifying the body with herbal supplements, it makes available vital medications formerly too difficult or expensive to widely administer, it decreases the individual and environmental hazards smoking by greatly facilitating the cessation of this pervasive habit. As you will see, these are only a few of the critical advancements made possible by DVT.

This book recognizes vaporization's synergistic relationship with natural and holistic approaches to the human body and mind, and advocates a return to the purity of nature which has been long eclipsed by Western Medical approaches and the synthesization of medicine. However, Vapor stands alone in that, in that unlike many texts which do so while attempting to depreciate the value of modern science and technology, Vapor instead embraces this technology and takes a refreshing look at how modern science and naturalistic approaches combine for a powerful advancement in human health and wellness.

Plants are our lifeblood and plant material offers us all the nutrients and remedies truly symbiotic with the human body. Digital Vaporization opens the door to a true integration of technology and holistic medicine. We are beginning to realize that synthesized does not inherently mean better, and that each individual must be evaluated in their own right and choose the therapy most beneficial to them.

One of the reasons vaporization is so exciting is that it allows each individual to become his or her own *phytotechnician*. Though we have long had the information and communication, we have lacked the necessary tools for the implementation of this approach.

The method of DVT is so recently perfected in fact, that even two years ago a successful device would not have been possible. The profound effects of this reach far into the current population. Its effect on the smoking industry alone will increase the health and longevity of millions. Though the full potential of vaporization won't be realized for perhaps another decade, it is happening right now.

You hold in your hands the very first book to be written on digital vaporization therapy. Years from now, you'll remember when you only first heard of vaporization and likely doubted its efficacy. Very few will yet have the foresight to realize its full range of possibility.

Shaahin Sean Cheyene
February, 2003

Contents

"The times, they are a-changin'..."
Bob Dylan

Introduction

Times are changing. People are changing and the ways that we take medicines, natural and synthetic alike, are also changing. Our current means of ingesting substances are soon to be obsolete. Inhalation technology is the hottest new frontier for the delivery of substances into the human body.

For millennia, people have used the technology of inhaling plant essences, alkaloids, and volatile elements in an effort to obtain their maximum benefits. Traditionally this has taken the form of either inhaling smoke or inhaling aromas from hot volatile oils such as those used in aromatherapy.

Many ancient civilizations, including the Chinese, Celts, Persians, and Romans, heated plant substances to release the volatile elements and aromas. Surprisingly, the smoke and aromatherapy techniques they used endured through thousands of years and resemble the methods in use today. Throughout the ages many cultures have developed a keen sense of the benefits of inhaling plant essences.

In Paleolithic times, evidence indicates that early man also burned plants in order to ward off evil spirits. In the sixteenth century, a physician by the name of Nostradamus, the infamous mystic and psychic whose predictions we recognize even today, was renowned for his miraculous aromatherapy techniques used to combat the plague. Native Americans burned mixtures of various plants in their rituals. History is filled with examples of civilizations and people using smoke, plants, and aromatherapy to various ends.

In modern times aromatherapy, smoke and new inhalation technologies abound. We are finding better ways to inhale medicines and new rituals to incorporate these valuable allies into our daily routines.

In the future, this inhalation technology will have the ability to ease the pain and suffering of millions, and it will be able to treat and prevent diseases. Inhalation technology will lead to the end of needles and the numerous diseases associated with their use. This technology will save the lives of millions and ease the lives of millions more.

Naturopathic doctors, holistic and alternative healthcare professionals, as well as medical doctors will be using inhalation technology with digital accuracy to treat patients.

This digital accuracy and the advent of better electronic technologies have opened the doorway to more advanced and better tools for inhalation technology.

In the future each person will possess the necessary tools to be their own phyto-technician. Each person will be able to quickly and easily use individualized plant combinations to aid their health and well-being. They will be empowered with the ability to inhale the true and active essence of a substance, such as a plant matter, without suffering the harmful byproducts associated with burning and smoking.

Inhaling plant aromas and other medicines is growing from a simple activity into a fine art and meticulous science. This book is the first and most basic comprehensive look at this technology. It will not be the last.

Read this book and take notes as you experiment. Develop your own techniques, medicines, devices, and improvements to what has been done in the past and share it with others for a more advanced future. It is my hope that each reader will generate unique and creative ideas about vaporization methods, applications, and benefits and share these ideas in order to propagate the awareness and use of vaporization technology. I believe each of us can play a part in taking this critical technology to its next level, increasing its significance and overall benefit to our daily lives. As this movement grows and people and technologies unite and emerge, the science and art of vaporization will grow and, with it, a better world and eventually the advancement of mankind.

Shaahin Sean Cheyene
Malibu, California
December, 2001

“Give me a lever long enough and a fulcrum on which to place it,
and I shall move the world.”
Archimedes, Pappus of Alexandria

1 WHAT IS VAPORIZATION?

From the microchip to polymer plastics to vaccinations to the World Wide Web — technological advancements achieved in the last century touch nearly every aspect of our lives. And yet we've only begun to realize the potential of such astounding progress in science, industry and medicine. Each advancement opens the door to new avenues of discovery, new possibilities for a higher quality of life. Undeniably, human beings in the 21st century enjoy more recreational and healthy-living choices than ever before.

Despite this ground swell of advancement, however, certain critical areas remain virtually untouched. Our methods of recreational drug delivery, most especially smoking, are one such example. Burning tobacco is an incredibly hazardous way to obtain the benefits of nicotine. Yet, until very recently no progress has been made in an alternate delivery system. Despite the past decade's considerable growth in the development of bio-engineered medications, our methods of delivering these or any substances to the body outside of a medically supervised environment remain limited and imprecise. For more on this, see the Addendum, but for now keep in mind that the hypodermic syringe predates the American Civil War and the first record of smoking is traced to the Mayans in 600 AD. Whether homeopathic remedies or synthesized medications, our current drug-delivery techniques are basic, archaic, and verging on obsolete.

Your doctor may deliver remedies via pills, syringes, skin patches, or particle inhalers. You may ingest herbal substances by swallowing raw or extracted plant material or by drinking tea brewed from suitable leaves. We can absorb certain effects through the skin by way of a poultice or salve, or we can inhale the desired essence through the smoke of the burning plant. Yet each of these methods has limitations and in some cases, outright dangers. It's been nearly four decades since technology has advanced enough to let us clearly see the hazards of taking a substance through the inhalation of its smoke; however, our advanced technologies have yet to be applied to an alternative method of viably delivering these substances directly from the plants themselves.

This is the 21st century! We can manufacture a *human heart*, yet we're chained to the carcinogenic byproducts of combustion in order to receive the desired herbal benefits.

Not any more.

This book will introduce you to process known as Phyto-Vaporization, or Phyto-

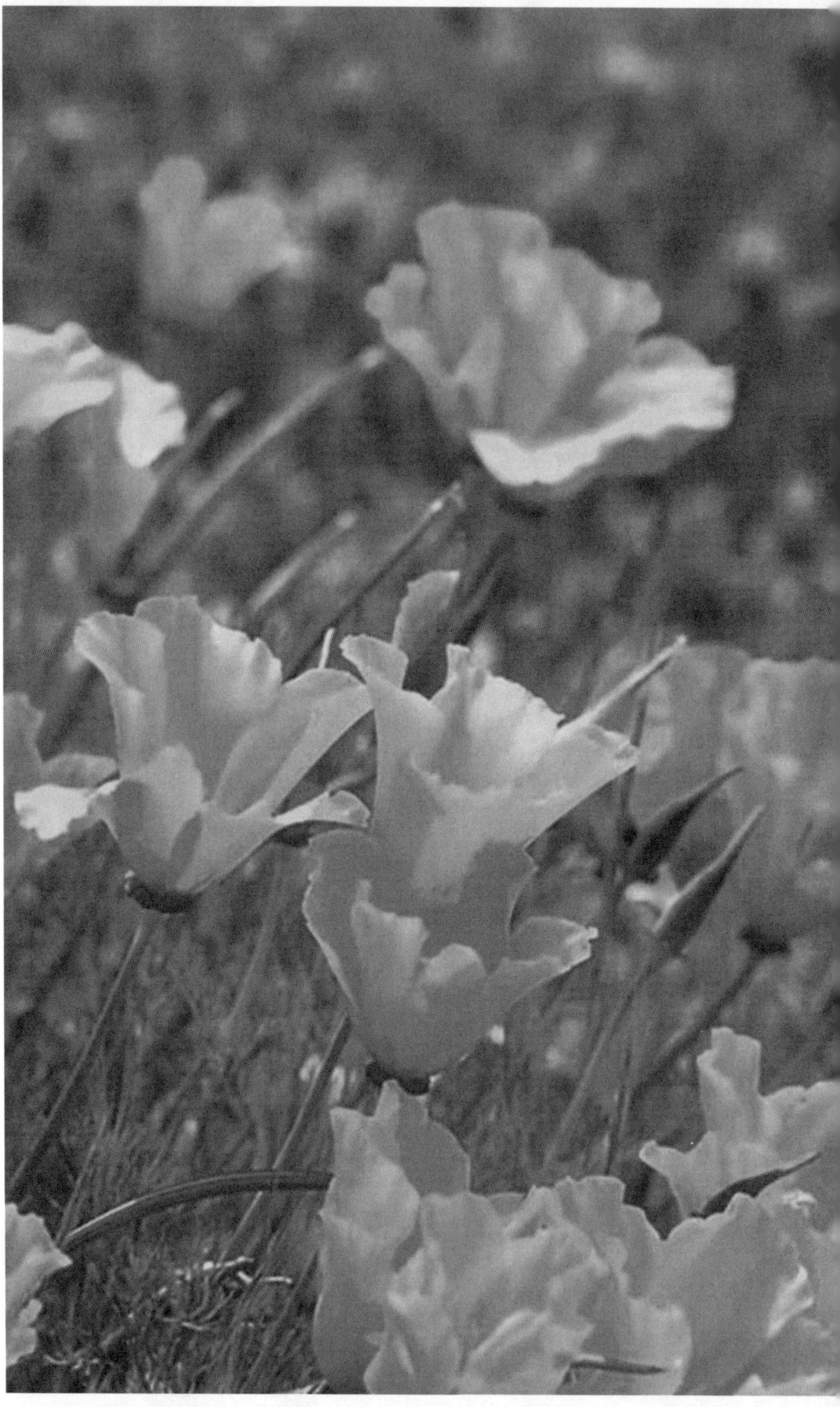

Inhalation (Phyto means "plant").

Vaporization is a substance delivery method purer than smoking, quicker and more direct than swallowing pills, and painless compared to needles. It is the new revolution in substance delivery and is poised to strengthen and enrich the medical, homeopathic, and smoking industries.

This book will explain how and why vaporization works, discuss the future implications of this method on the homeopathic, tobacco, and medical industries, and give you an overview of helpful herbs and how to use them. When you finish this book you'll be on your way to learning the ways you can benefit from this truly revolutionary process, and have the preliminary tools you need to take charge of your health and become your own phyto-technician.

First, let's take a closer look at science of vaporization.

VAPORIZATION DEFINED

Vaporization, also known as volatization, is a process by which the active elements of a substance are released through the application of heat *without combustion*. In other words, the substance is heated, but never burned.

This is an important distinction because when a substance is burned it becomes *denatured*. Denaturing means that a chemical change takes place and the molecular structure of the substance is actually modified. When denaturing is catalyzed by excessive heat this is known as *pyrolysis*. Pyrolysis is a major drawback to smoking a material. When pyrolysis occurs, a molecular breakdown creates new elements that had not been present in the source material prior to combustion.

The obvious example is, of course, tobacco. When smoking a cigarette, you seek the effects of tobacco's active element, nicotine. Through the process of smoking, however, you receive not only nicotine, but a handful of toxins and irritants, such as smoke and tar, which have been created by pyrolysis. In contrast, because vaporization typically requires a temperature lower than a substance's combustion point, pyrolysis never takes place and the substance is never denatured. In other words, vaporization releases the active elements of a substance through a method by which pyrolysis cannot take place. Therefore, it produces a pure aerosol mist comprised only of elements naturally occurring in the source material.

THE KEY TO VAPORIZATION

The key to vaporization is *temperature*: digitally precise, accurately maintained temperature.

Vaporization is also known as volatization because it releases the volatile elements in a substance. In herbs, these are mostly the oils.

Scientists discovered the temperature at which the active elements in a plant will evaporate and aerosolize can be lower than the temperature at which that plant will combust. If correctly applied, a lower temperature will cause the release of an herb's essential elements into an inhalable steam and, provided the heat source remains at the lower temperature, the substance will never be burned.

No smoke. No smoky odor. Just pure vapor from the botanical mixture of your choice.

From Plant to Vapor?

Let's take a moment to discuss what's actually happening with vaporization. We all understand the concept of liquid to solid or liquid to gas — boiling water and freezing ice are examples we see every day. But solid to gas is a bit more difficult to picture.

All plants are imbued with oils that hold many of the desired elements for a medicine or homeopathic remedy. For example, in the case of aromatherapy, a chamomile leaf contains a center layer of essential oils. In fact, these oils contain the aroma and therapeutic benefits of the herb. The oils in each plant type will boil at a temperature specific to that plant. Boiling points depend mainly on the density of the oil. When the liquid within the leaves — the oil — begins to boil, the molecules will move more quickly, and spread farther apart. It is this action which thins the density of the oil from a heavier-than-air liquid, to a lighter-than-air gas. The substance can then be pulled by air and inhaled into the lung. In mist form, the particles of the oil are small enough to be absorbed into the alveoli (tiny air sacs that cover the surface of the lower lung) where they are almost immediately taken into the blood stream.

As the vaporization continues, the essential oils are lifted from the plant ,and it becomes curled, and withered. It may darken in color and will often leave behind only a clean, dry, and crumbled substance.

Benefits of Vaporization

Let's compare the health effects of consumption via vaporization, ingestion, and smoking.

The vast majority of herbs today are enjoyed by ingestion. Supplements may be taken in pill form, brewed into teas, or by simply eating the plant itself. The active ingredients of the plant, however, must pass through a series of obstacles that may degrade the plant's active elements before finally entering the blood stream and benefiting the user. However, as digestive enzymes break down herbal remedies, they degrade their effect and sometimes even catalyze a change in the material. In addition, a time delay of noticeable effect often makes proper dosing a problem. Ingestion is a relatively safe, but significantly inefficient way to benefit from herbs and medicines.

Inhalation is another choice and the most common form of this is smoking. Tobacco has been used for thousands of years. Millions of people have enjoyed the plant as an herbal aid, a religious and ritualistic device, and for recreational enjoyment. Over the past 30 years we have finally developed the technology and medical advances to recognize the health dangers inherent in the combustion of this or any herb. Yet few herbal delivery options have been developed to replace combustion.

Over the next few years, vaporization promises to be a prominent alternative to current methods of drug delivery and aromatherapy.

General Health Benefits of Vaporization

• Vaporization produces no combustion byproducts such as carbon monoxide, tar or other carcinogenic elements.
• Vapor is considerably cooler than smoke and less likely to damage lung tissue.
• Vaporization provides a purer, more concentrated effect and requires less of the substance than if smoked or ingested.
• The substance is not degraded by digestive acids before entering the blood.
• There are no fillers or buffers as with pills.
• Vaporization acts quickly. The substance enters bloodstream more quickly than most methods.
• There is no danger of contaminated needles as in injections.
• Digital precision and the rapid onset of effect help to establish an exact dose specific to each user.

The potential impact of digital vaporization is enormous. On a consumer level, over the next few years, digital vaporization will revolutionize both the aromatherapy and smoking cessation industries. On a pharmaceutical level, medical vaporization will significantly enhance the industries of drug delivery, dietary supplements, pharmaceuticals, biotech, and defense.

Future generations will marvel at our barbaric practices of inhaling smoke and piercing our skin to receive medication. But before we gaze into the future, let's first take a look at the past.

"Smell is a potent wizard which transports us across time
and all the years we have lived."
Helen Keller

2 AROMATHERAPY THROUGHOUT THE AGES

Healing Through the Sense of Scents

Vaporization deals extensively with the inhalation of essential plant oils. In this way, it is kindred with aromatherapy, and poised to dramatically enhance this growing practice. For this reason, we'll take a look at man's recognition and experimentation with essential oils over the centuries.

As with the dawn of herbal medicine, the beginnings of aromatherapy are difficult to specify. We do know that essential oils such as olive, castor, and sesame, which could be extracted by pressure, rather than the more complex and modern distillation method, were used in the East during the Neolithic period 6,000 - 9,000 years ago.

3,000 – 2,000 BC

Artifacts unearthed in ancient Egypt have included ointment containers and alabaster pots highly suggestive of aromatic use. The Egyptians enjoyed a sophisticated cultural life, to be unparalleled by any, even by those to whom their civilization fell, for thousands of years. In addition to highly developed mathematics, literature, and art, the Egyptians enjoyed refinements such as jewelry, cosmetics, and beatification products. Perfumes were popular, often in the form of an unguent, or thick salve, which was applied to the top of the head on men and women alike. The unguent would slowly melt and bathe the user in aromatic oils throughout the day.

In addition, the essential oils of myrrh and cedar wood were among those used in the intricate process of mummification, and modern science has confirmed myrrh's antiseptic and anti-bacterial properties, and has proved cedar wood oil to be a strong fixative agent. At the time, as throughout the ages, medicine and religion were inextricably bound. The first true "aromatherapists" were holy men such as priests who would dispense oils for medicinal and spiritual purification rituals.

Egyptian temples would burn frankincense and various gums and resins in an attempt to clear worshippers' minds and promote focused meditation and purity of thought.

Heliopolis, Egypt's "City of the Sun", faithfully appeased the Sun God Ra by burning resins in the morning, myrrh at noon, and *kyphi* at sunset. Kyphi, perhaps the most notorious of all Egyptian fragrances, was believed to induce hypnotic states. The name

Kyphi — Aroma for the Gods

Kyphi is an ancient Egyptian ceremonial incense made from various resins, herbs and spices. Kyphis is seeped in wine, honey and essential oils. Kyphi was burned through the night to appease Ra, the Sun God and to bring good fortune. The Greek philosopher Plutrach said of the mesmerizing power of kyphi: "Its aromatic substances lull to sleep, allay anxieties, and brighten dreams. It is made of things that delight most in the night and exhibits its virtues by night."

Ingredients were believed to be linked to specific powers, such as:

Jasmine ~ *Luck in love*
Musk ~ *Inciting sexual desire*
Copal ~ *Easing tension after a quarrel*
Lavender ~ *Easing heartbreak*
Bergamot ~ *Attracting money*
Red Ginger ~ *Success and improvement*
Frankincense ~ *Protection and strength*

Try this traditional Egyptian kyphi recipe. It makes an excellent incense ball and lasts for years. (courtesy of www.herbalmusings.com)

Place ¼ cup raisins in a bowl. Add just enough white wine to cover the raisins, cover loosely with a tea towel or cheesecloth, and allow to steep for seven days. On the third day, blend equal parts of the following powdered herbs in a bit of white wine: Juniper, Acacia, Henna, Sweet Sedge Root. After two days, drain and reserve any liquid. On the last day, drain the raisin mixture, reserving the liquid. In a small bowl mix together equal parts of the following ground herbs: Calamus, Gum Mastic, Peppermint, Bay Laurel, Orris, Cinnamon, and Galangal. Set aside. In another small bowl, blend together 1 Tbls. powdered myrrh, and 1 Tbls. clove honey. To this mixture add the ground herbs, and the raisins and herbs steeped in wine. Blend well. Add a little of the reserved wine if the mixture becomes too dry. Shape into ⅝" balls and roll balls in benzoin. Lay out on waxed paper for a week or so, until firm. For best results, let cure for 2 – 3 weeks.

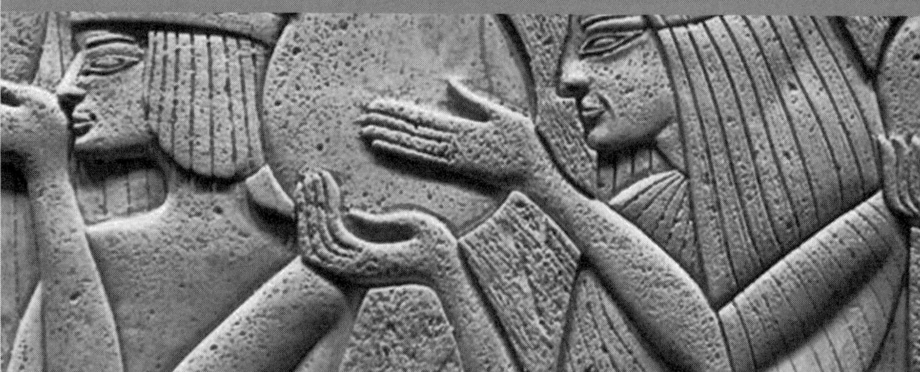

kyphi translates literally to "welcome to the gods". This herb was renowned for its ability to encourage sleep, quell anxiety, enhance dreaming, alleviate sorrow, and act as an overall elixir against toxins. Kyphi is still in use today.

A Babylonian tablet from 1,800 BC revealed an order for a large quantity of "imported oil of cedar, myrrh, and cypress". This suggests not only advanced techniques of wood-pressing extraction, but also a 4,000-year-old international trade of aromatic oils.

1,240 BC

The Bible, whether taken as literature, historical text, or Holy Word, has numerous significant references to essential plant oils. Moses, during the exodus from Egypt, was instructed to make holy oil and incense from myrrh, cinnamon, sweet calamus, and olive oil. Certain perfumes were considered so sacred that their misuse would result in exile. The New Testament contains frequent mentions of anointing, including this passage from the Last Supper:

> Mary, therefore, having taken a pound of ointment of pure nard of great price, anointed the feet of Jesus, and wiped his feet with her hair, and the house was filled with the odour of the ointment. –*John 12:3*

Furthermore, the basement of a dwelling in Jerusalem from 1 BC revealed evidence of a perfumery that likely supplied a nearby temple.

7 AD

Chinese Taoists have long believed the extraction of a plant's essential oils and fragrance represent the liberation of its soul. The single word *heang* holds the Chinese meaning for perfume, incense, and fragrance. Heang has been divided into six categories according to the mood evoked by the substance. Roughly translated, these basic classifications are: tranquil, reclusive, luxurious, beautiful, refined, and noble.

The seventh century saw the onset of the Tang dynasties, though which the noble class made extravagant uses of fragrance for the next one thousand years. Lavishly fragrance baths, clothing, temples, paper, ink, delicate wooden fans, and scent-filled sachets permeated high-society China. The Silk Route through Asia brought the Chinese imported jasmine, rose water, cloves, ginger and patchouli.

400 – 1,500 AD

During the Middle Ages in Europe, aromatics were often employed against the recurring plagues. Pine wood was burned in the streets to fumigate the area. These fires would be re-fueled every twelve hours in an effort to protect against the airborne poison or "aura" of the disease. Countless aromatic substances were used in various forms to combat Black Death, including perfumed candles in sick rooms. We now know that all aromatics possess antiseptic properties so it makes sense that close contact with airborne aromatic oils were likely protected, to varying degrees, from the disease.

Until the 19th Century, in fact, medical practitioners would carry aromatics in a small perforated box, known as a cassolette, atop their walking sticks. They would hold the cassolette to their noses when treating especially contagious patients.

1,900s Aromatherapy

The French chemist René-Maurice Gattefossé, who began his studies with the cosmetic applications of essential oils, grew to be known as the father of modern aromatherapy. He realized the medicinal capabilities of essential oils after a laboratory accident in which his right hand was severely burned. He immersed the wound in the nearest liquid, which happened to be lavender oil. Amazed by the ease and speed of recovery from the burn, Gattefossé immediately began to study the properties and benefits of essential oils. He eventually coined the phrase aromatherapy and taught that "the whole is greater than the sum of its parts", advocating use of natural substances in their entirety. His first book, *Aromathérapie*, published in 1928, stirred much interest in the field.

Fifteen years later, Jean Valet, a medical doctor, began treating patients with essential oils while working as a surgeon during World War II. Though supplies were scarce, Valet found that essential oils often provided valuable relief to the wounded. His 1964 publication, also entitled *Aromathérapie*, helped establish the discipline of aromatherapy in the modern world.

Around this time, the work of Italian Drs. Gatti and Cajola studied both the medical and psychological applications of aromatherapy. More recently, Paolo Rovesti, of the Instituo Derivati Vegetali in Milan, began clinically establishing and documenting the effects of these essential oils.

Current

Today, aromatherapy is used throughout the world. Science continues to support the long-held physical and psychological benefits of aromatherapy. Once relegated to the realm of "alternative" medicine, aromatherapy and holistic practices are slowly rising in status and becoming recognized as a valuable compliment to conventional western medicine.

Whether lighting a scented candle, taking a fragrant bath, using a scented lotion, or walking through a bloom-filled garden, we are affected every day by the essential oils of plants. The focused and purposeful application of those essences is the root of this widely popular practice.

WHAT IS AROMATHERAPY?

Aromatherapy promotes the health and well-being of the body and mind through the use of the essential oils of plants. These potent oils offer an incredible arsenal against illness and disharmony in the body. Aromatherapy combines holistic techniques with the application of essential oils to enhance the quality of life both physically and psychologically. In contrast to synthetic drugs, essential oils, although powerful and acutely effective, do not linger and leave toxins in the body.

Essential oils, when inhaled, invigorate and stimulate a healing or healthful state.

Principles

Aromatherapy is a holistic practice. This means it regards the body as a total organism, a complex system of opposing forces which, rather than examining individual symptoms, must be treated as a whole. Aromatherapy is based on a set of complimentary principals of nature and life. These principals are founded in the concept of balance and harmony both within and between life systems. Though subtle variations exist between each individual, Robert Tissand, in his book *The Art of Aromatherapy*, outlines three overriding concepts.

Life Force

To the Chinese it is *ch'i*, for the Indians *pranna*, but no matter what the term, life force is the vital energy which drives and enforces all life. It binds the elements of an atom, it sustains the pull of gravity and magnetism, it causes a plant to push forth from the dirt and bloom, and it gives us the very consciousness to ponder its existence. Aromatherapists believe that the essential oil of a plant is akin to its life force, which is extremely delicate. If excessively tampered with, the life force and value of the essence, and of the essential oil, may be lost. Plants are most beneficial in their whole and unaltered state. The organic nature of plant essences is what allows it to work in such powerful harmony with the body.

Life force is a ubiquitous energy that constantly strives for a state of health and harmony. Consider, for instance, the duality and balance of body systems such as blood pressure, respiration, cardiac function, and the equilibrium of chemicals in our very cells. Our neurons fire based on the balance of pH levels, which in turn are regulated by the relation and balance of elements within and without the cell wall.

The pervading struggle for equilibrium in the body tells us we cannot force ourselves to heal. Rather, we can encourage healing through the promotion of balance and harmony.

Yin and Yang

From the Chinese, we get the principal of yin and yang, which are the two opposing energies in every life force. Everything has both yin and yang properties and a change of predominance from one to the other is a matter of subtle flow, a slow shift of balance. Understanding which essential oils are primarily yin or yang will help determine their application in treating an illness or imbalance in the body. Yin is associated with sedation and has a cooling effect, while yang represents stimulation and heating.

Organic Foods

Whole foods, natural and unrefined, are the basis for a healthy and balanced body system. Natural foods are in perfect proportion intrinsically. Adding or subtracting from

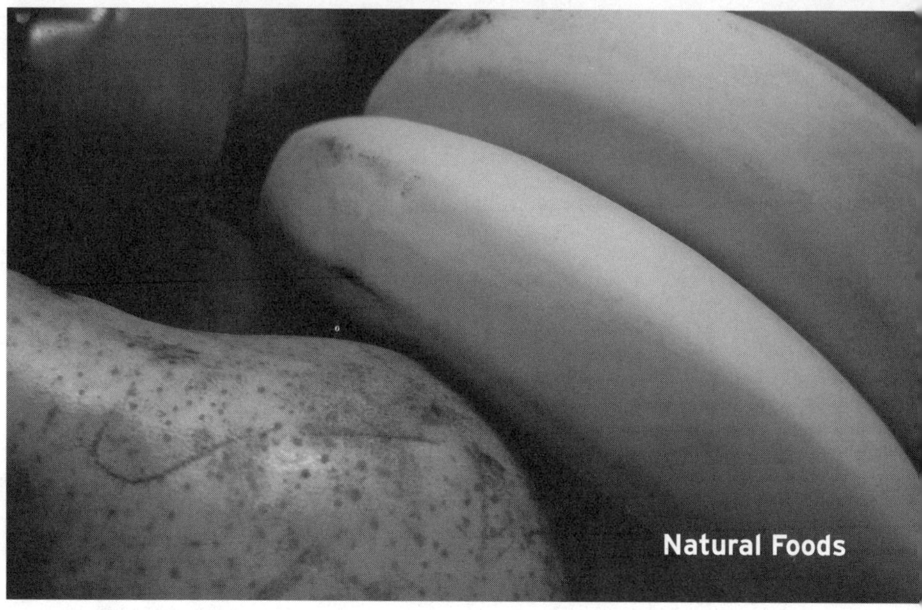

natural foods only upsets this balance and adds to malnutrition, taxes the body, and promotes general ill health. The very same problem applies to synthetically altered forms of medicine. Negative side effects display the body's desire to purge the offensive substance, which may be intended to treat a specific symptom, but disrupts the body as a whole. The use of highly refined foods, such as bleached flour and sugar and synthetic medicines, over time, will hinder liver and metabolic function, drain energy from the body, and weaken its natural ability to heal. A healthy, organic diet consists of fresh fruits and vegetables, grains such as rice, whole wheat, and oats, and a limited amount of high-protein foods.

HOW DOES AROMATHERAPY WORK?

Olfactory Anatomy — "The Nose Knows"

Our sense of smell is one of our most basic instincts. In early human evolution our sense of smell was vital, more so even than our sight. Scent gave important information about our environment and the animals and humans around us.

Physiologically, evidence of this connection remains. There is only one place in the human body where the central nervous system comes into direct contact with the environment and this is at the olfactory membrane. Information from the nerve cells travels directly to the limbic system, which is one of the most primal areas of the brain. The limbic system is associated with base memory, instinct, and emotional and sexual impulses.

All other sensory information enters the brain through the thalamus. This means, for example, that you are able to see and cognitively recognize an object almost simultaneously. With olfactory information, however, your body may experience and *chemically react* to a scent before you are even aware the scent exists. It is this most basic and direct input into the body which makes scent such a powerful memory stimulant and healing agent.

Aromatherapy Techniques

Vaporization eliminates the needs for these extraction techniques, as the process itself releases the volatile elements, the essential oils, directly and naturally from the plant itself. Oil may also be extracted by these alternate methods:

Expression — This was likely the first method used for the extraction of essential oils. Today, expression is primarily used for citrus fruits. Oils are isolated by pressure; they are literally squeezed from sacs in the rind or peel of the fruit.

Steam Distillation — This is the most common form of distillation. Steam passes through the plant matter, heating and releasing the essential oils. The water from the steam and the oils are collected together and then separated. The oil is collected and stored for later use, rather than freshly inhaled. This method is usually performed commercially.

Enfleurage — From the French "in flowers", this method goes back nearly a century and is based on the discovery that essential plant oils are soluble in fat. Plant matter is seeped in a fatty substance, sometimes a vegetable oil. Leached plants are continually replaced until the fat is rich with essential oil. The fat is then dissolved with an alcohol-based solvent, leaving only the essential oil.

Solvent Extraction — This has come to replace enfleurage with a method of seeping plant material directly in an alcohol solvent that produces a waxy paste. This paste is then seeped in pure alcohol, which dissolves the wax. The remaining liquid is known as an "absolute".

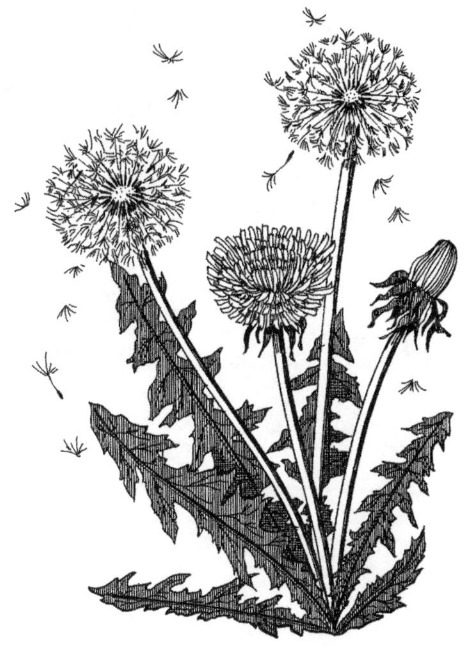

No matter how extracted, these volatile oils can be used to soothe a variety of stresses and ailments. Often used in conjunction with massage therapy, stress reduction, and organic diet, inhaling these vital plant essences will help restore balance and vitality to the body.

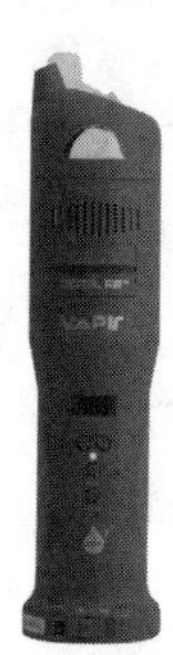

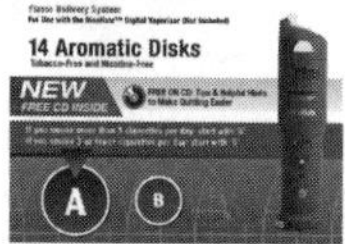
NicoHale
The Natural Way
14 Aromatic Disks
NEW
FREE CD INSIDE
A
B

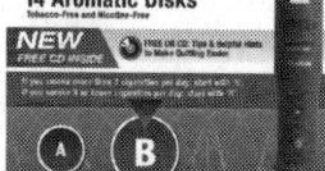
NicoHale
The Natural Way
14 Aromatic Disks
NEW
FREE CD INSIDE
A
B

3 THE CURRENT MARKET OF VAPORIZATION PRODUCTS

Search the Internet and you'll find dozens of sites peddling different forms of so- called "vaporizer" products. Many attempt to offer a quick and inexpensive means for the average consumer to vaporize herbs in their home. But look closely. The devices often employ crude heating methods. A surprising number of "vaporizers" use an assortment of glass domes and remote heating devices such as a heat gun, soldering iron, or open flame. Some are little more than a heat source, rubber hose, and mason jar, and almost none provide the vaporization benefits discussed in this book. Here's why:

Remember pyrolysis? When a constant temperature is not maintained, a substance may heat beyond its vaporization point and begin to burn. Because these devices have no means of temperature control, the substances will heat to their vaporization point and beyond — producing vaporized mist for a few seconds and quickly moving into combustion. Conversely, a temperature that cools to below the vaporization point, before all of an herb's active elements have been released, will result in a wet residue and wasted herbs. Efforts to prevent such waste result in sheer guesswork as the user experiments with applying the heat source for different amounts of time and at different distance from the source material. Given that each substance has its own vaporization temperature and rate, this is an imperfect system at best.

Although marketed as vaporizers, most of these devices are ineffective and little more than an alternate means of smoking. And worse, some of these heat guns and soldering irons actually *come into contact* with the material and char it directly. If the material is in direct contact with the heating element, the heating element heats very quickly and during the time it takes for it to cool, it actually burns the material. Additionally, these devices are often made of industrial grade metals which can release toxins into the vapor stream. Food-grade ceramic is the safest heating element for vaporization. Be sure to exercise extreme caution when shopping for a vaporizer and select only vaporizers with food grade ceramic heating elements.

Currently, very few companies produce respectable, consumer-grade vaporizers. Use the following comparison as a guide in your search for the vaporizer which best suits your needs.

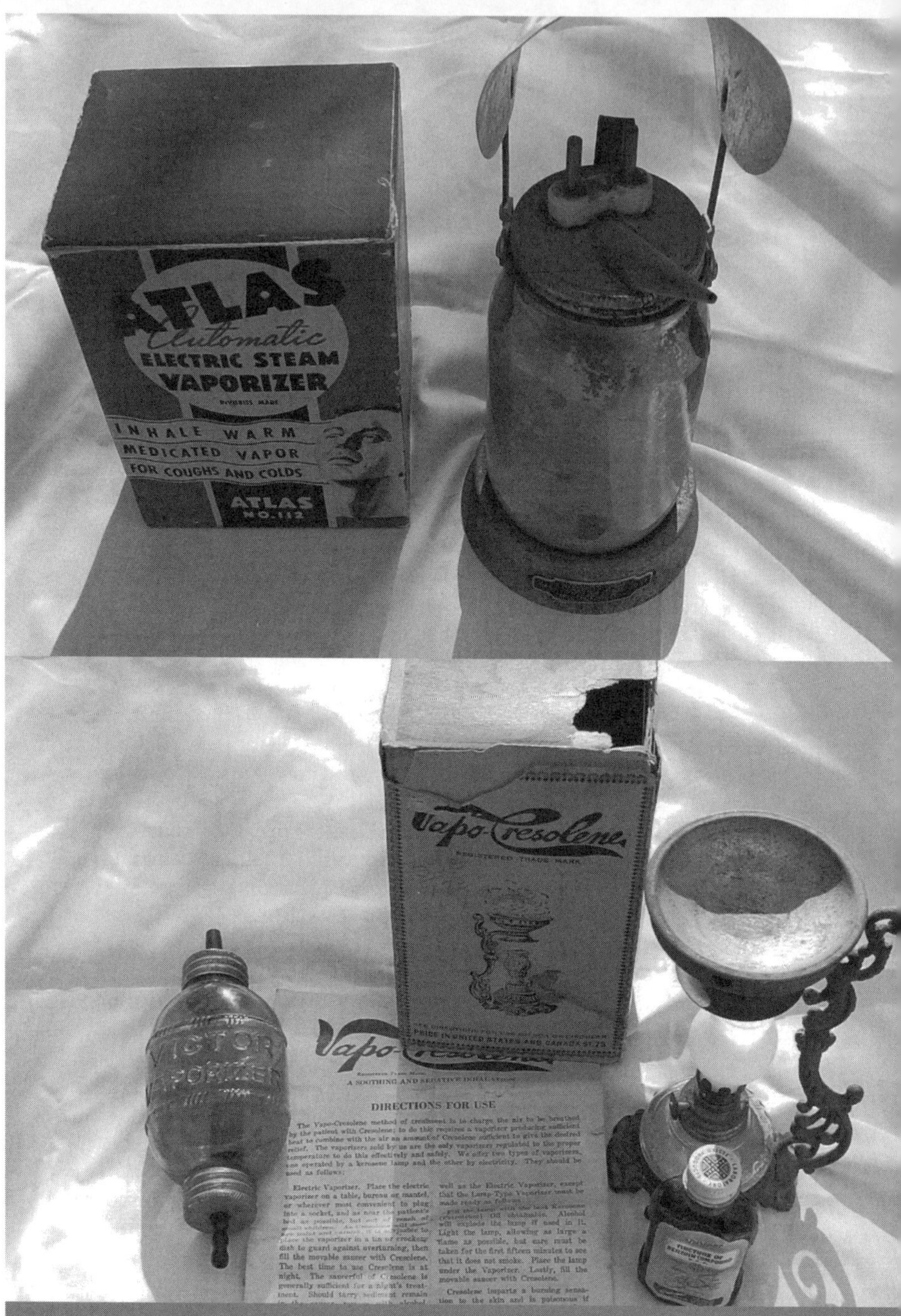

An assortment of old vaporizing devices. All of them burn the material, and none are capable of maintaining a constant, controllable temperature for vaporization.

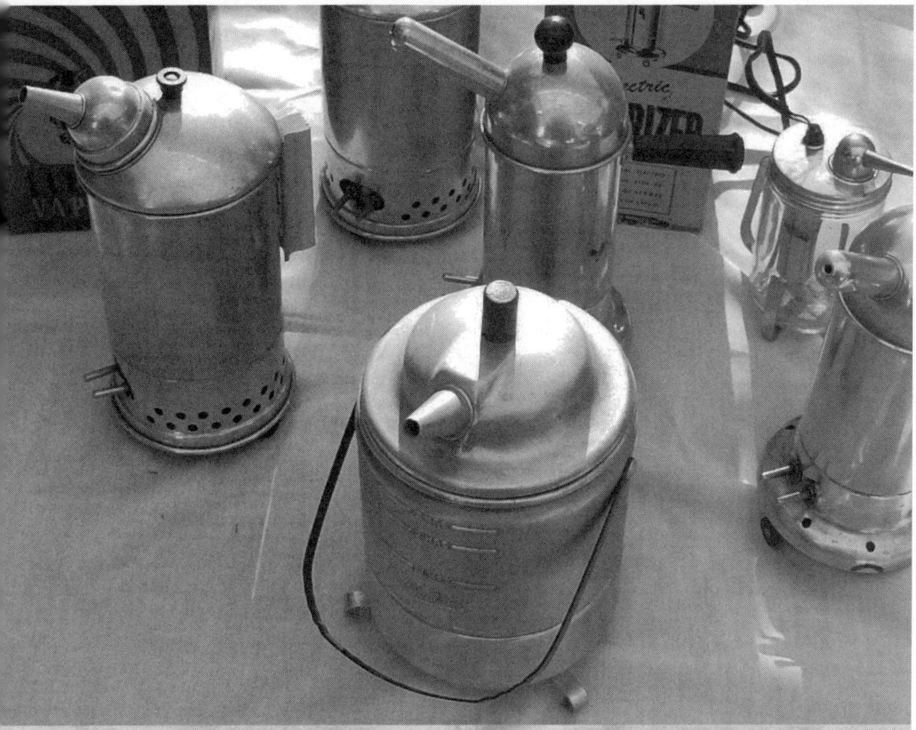

PE-PO

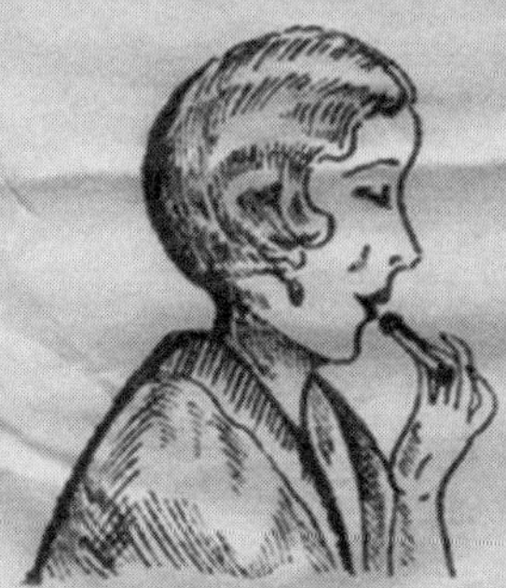

**İNHA-
LATOR**

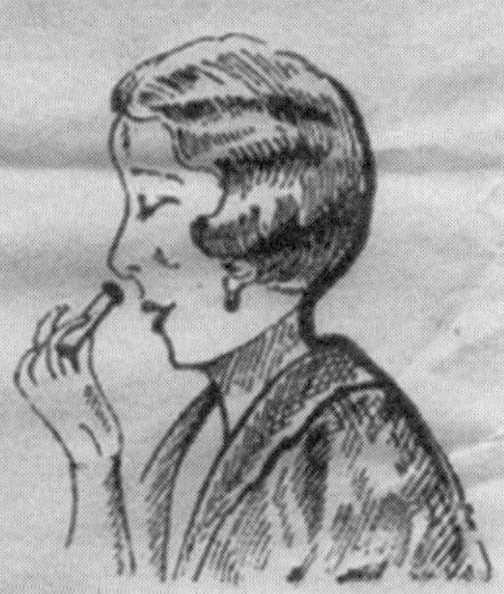

Teneffüs yollarını açar, Sinirleri teskin ve serinlendirir, Soğuk algınlıklıkları uzaklaştırır

CLASS I: DIGITAL VAPORIZATION

I must admit that my work in vaporization over the years has led me to create a company, Advanced Inhalation Revolutions, Inc., or AIR2, that is developing and marketing the only digital vaporizer available today. I truly believe that this product is the best there is, but I would be remiss in not mentioning my involvement with the company and technology development. You can make your own judgment.

This class of vaporizer offers the highest quality manufacturing and the most sophisticated technological control over the vaporization process. Digital temperature regulation is the most effective method to prevent partial combustion of the material. Only one vaporizer currently offers digital vaporization.

Company: Advanced Inhalation Revolutions, Inc. (AIR2)
Device: Vapir

This company currently produces the most advanced consumer-level vaporizer on the market. Herbs fit into a mesh disk that slides into the unit. Temperature and time are both digitally controlled and the unit maintains temperature via a closed-loop thermostat. Material is never burned, there is no assembly and no danger of overheating the substance. Advanced Inhalation Revolutions, Inc. also offers the only battery-powered vaporizer in the world. The cordless model adds new freedom to the vaporization experience as the unit is fully portable.

Strengths:

- No assembly required, compact, simple to use.
- Fully portable. Device is available with high-powered battery, and D/C adapters for use in an airplane and car.
- Mesh disks are the simplest method of herb vaporization to date and are unique to the product.
- Digital technology maintains constant temperature; therefore, herbs cannot be overheated. Highly accurate.
- Wide assortment of accessories to enhance vaporiza-

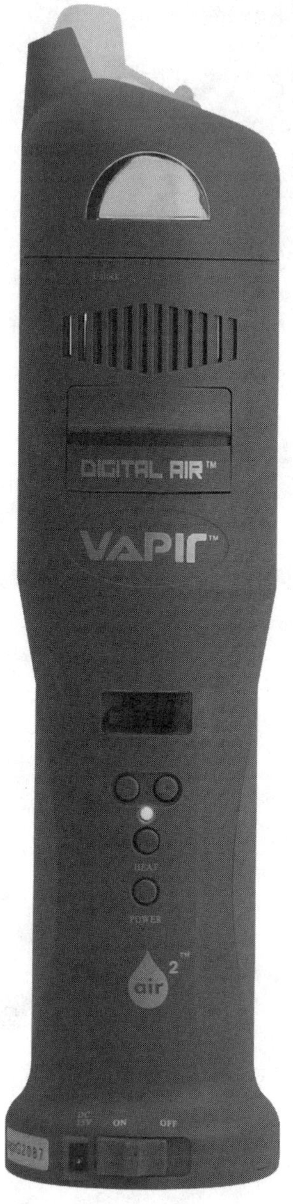

A Vapir digital vaporizer, photo courtesy of AIR2

tion experience.
• Corded and Cordless models are both available.

Weaknesses: —

Battery: Only lasts for one 25-minute vaporization session.
Price: $299 Basic, $399 Deluxe Re-Chargeable
Warranty: 90 days, parts and labor with an optional 3-year replacement plan.
Accessories: 10-pack of empty Herb Disks, back-pack carrying case, airplane charger, car charger, cigarette tube attachment, e-herbs flavored herbal moisturizer, e-herbs throat spray, organic cleaning liquid and brush, rechargeable lithium ion battery, reusable mesh materials holder, USB upgrade and USB cable, assortment of pre-packaged e-herbs on disk, NicoHale smoking cessation disks.

CLASS II: MANUALLY ADJUSTABLE TEMPERATURE

This class offers a means of manually adjusting temperature through electrical controls. These products do not self-maintain temperature and the danger of combustion remains present.

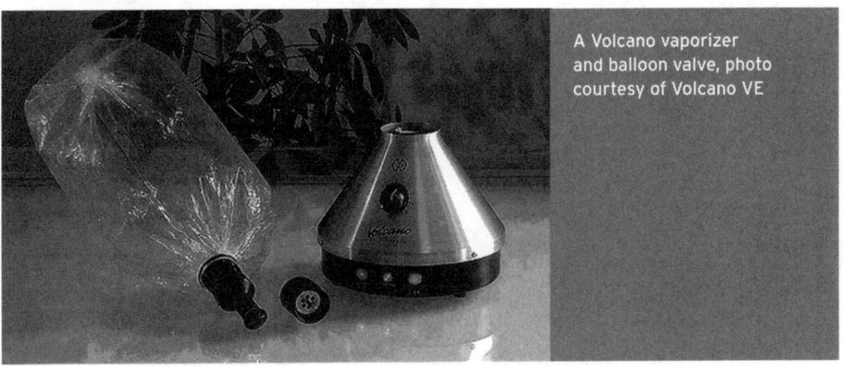

A Volcano vaporizer and balloon valve, photo courtesy of Volcano VE

Company: Volcano VE
Device: Volcano

The Volcano vaporizer utilizes a patented balloon valve to trap vapor prior to inhalation. The balloon then detaches from the unit and allows users to move about and inhale the vapor at their leisure. Constant airflow maintains temperature.

Strengths:
• High-grade materials. Excellent German workmanship.
• Unique, detachable, balloon vapor-collection chamber.
• Automated airflow.

Weaknesses:
• No digital temperature control.
• It is inconvenient and is not portable or rechargeable.
• Elements may be trapped in balloon and wasted.
• High price.
• According to the manufacturer, the Volcano is not available in the US due to its lack of proper safety approvals.

Price: \$400 – \$500
Warranty: 2-year warranty
Accessories: Replacement filters, multiple size balloon sets.

Company: Research and Experience
Device: Aromed Vaporizer

This company provides a digitally controlled device with a halogen-light heat source that connects to a glass bowl.

Strengths:
• Simple, easy to use.
• Digital Temperature Control.
• Great Post-Industrial rough design. (Could have been made by a mad scientist in his garage or laboratory!)
• Moderately effective.

Weaknesses:
• Many heating variables including: no constant airflow — vaporization is affected by the strength of user's air intake, which may raise or lower temperature.
• The unit is bulky and quite large.
• It is inconvenient, and not portable or rechargeable.
• It uses water to cool and filter vapor. Active ingredients may be absorbed by the water and never reach the lungs.
• Uneven heating. Light heats the surface of the materials unevenly. Requires constant mixing of herbs in bowl for even vaporization.
Price: \$330 – \$499 (depending on the distributor).
Warranty: none
Accessories: Carrying kit, replacement parts.

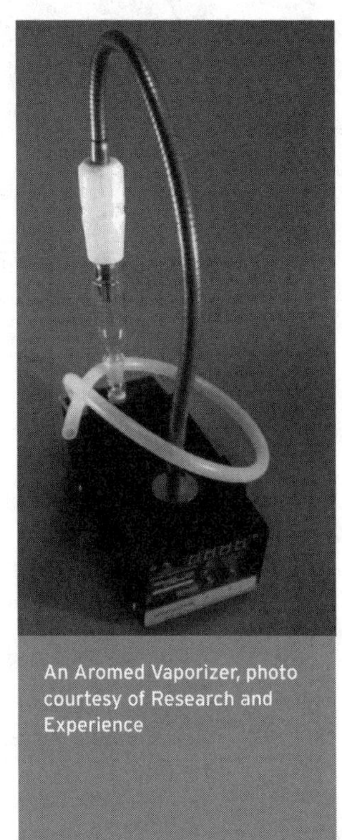
An Aromed Vaporizer, photo courtesy of Research and Experience

CLASS III: VAPORIZATION BY REMOTE HEATING DEVICE

This class uses a separate heating element such as a heat gun or specially designed heating "wand". The best of these models offers a heating device with incremental temperature control; most however, have a constant and un-regulated heat source. These products offer little control over herb temperature, and the danger of combustion is relatively high.

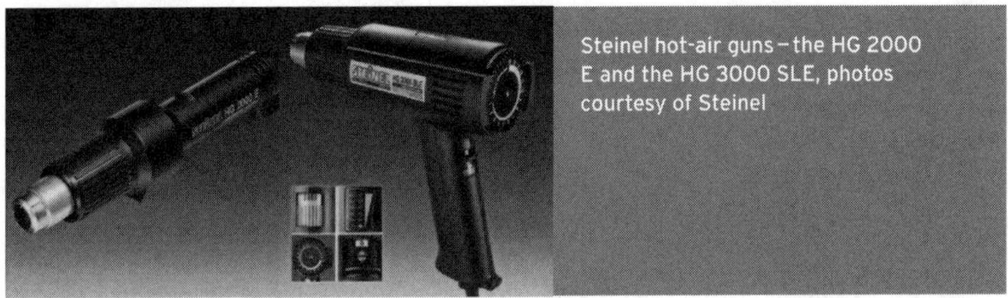

Steinel hot-air guns—the HG 2000 E and the HG 3000 SLE, photos courtesy of Steinel

Company: Steinel
Device: HG series hot-air gun

Although they don't actually sell a "vaporizer" *per se*, Steinel offers an effective "do-it-yourself" kit. This kit includes the top-of-the-line Steinel model HG 3002 LCD heat gun. Although the Steinel is the premiere heat gun currently available, keep in mind that this and all heat guns are designed for harsh tasks such as paint stripping, rather than the delicate process of vaporization. Steinel's home assembly approach is fairly popular, and if done properly is moderately effective. You may purchase parts from the company directly, or use their model to assemble your own.

Strengths:

- Temperate dial allows for more control than methods that use a less sophisticated heat-gun.
- Heat source does not come into contact with material.
- Effective.

Weaknesses:

- Difficult to assemble, must purchase several parts.
- Requires careful herb preparation and packing.
- The kit is bulky and requires intensive set up.
- Expensive.

• Inconvenient.
• Not portable or rechargeable.

Price: $420 for all the inclusive Vaporization Kit. Items may also be purchased individually.
Warranty: 90 days, parts and labor.
Accessories: All initial and replacement items may be purchased separately. Replacement parts kits also available.

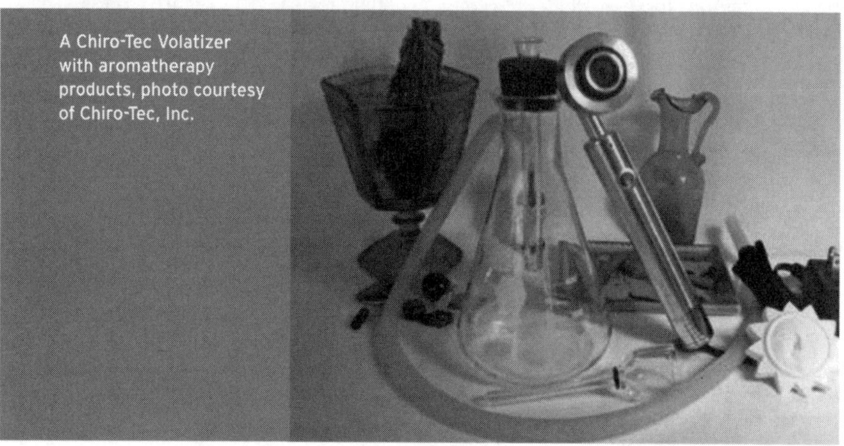
A Chiro-Tec Volatizer with aromatherapy products, photo courtesy of Chiro-Tec, Inc.

Company: Chiro-Tec, Inc.
Device: Volatizer: Models M1 and M2 "Black Beauty"

Although this product claims to use a method of vaporization or volatization, it refers to its device not as a vaporizer but as a "a rapid-onset, hot air extraction inhalant device". The Volatizer uses a water bowl system and comes with a glass jar, rubber hose and metal heating wand.

Strengths:
• Price flexibility. Aside from the heating wands, many parts may be purchased separately from local merchants.
• Soothing. Water flask eases throat irritation.
• Moderately effective.

Weaknesses:
• The largest drawback to this and all similar devices is the tendency to *burn* the materials. The heating wand has no means of regulating or even monitoring the temperature of the herbs. Only guesswork avoids partial burning.
• Additional heating variables such as no constant airflow — vaporization is affected by

the strength of the user's air intake, which may raise or lower the temperature.
• It is inconvenient and not portable or rechargeable.
• Available only in the US and Canada.

Price: $199 for Complete M2 Black Beauty. Parts may be purchased individually.
Warranty: None.
Accessories: An adapter for use with the heat gun, carrying case, replacement parts.

In addition to consumer-grade vaporizers, the pharmaceutical industry is developing medical-grade devices as well. We will go into these as we discuss the medical application of vaporization technology in the Addendum. For now, there is one major industry we have yet to address.

As you might expect, with the potential impact vaporization holds over the smoking industry, tobacco companies are themselves in the race to develop and control the ultimate consumer vaporizer product.

"In all things of nature there is something of the marvelous."
Aristotle (384 BC – 322 BC), *Parts of Animals*

4 VAPORIZATION AND HERBAL MEDICINE

WHAT IS AN HERB?

It seems like a simple question, but defining an herb is complicated. The *Oxford English Dictionary* defines an herb as "a term applied to plants where the leaves, or stems and leaves, are used for food or medicine, or in some way for their scent or flavor." This may seem inclusive, but this definition omits integral plants such as ginger, fennel, and ginseng. Obviously the roots, rhizome, seeds, and bark may be equally beneficial and designate an herb. If we broaden this definition beyond "leaves or stems and leaves" to include any part of a plant "used for food or medicine or in some way for its scent or flavor", the definition remains imprecise. Consider lettuce, for example. Is lettuce an herb? When consumed for lunch in a sandwich, no. However, wild lettuce, *Lactuca virosa*, is a mild sedative, analgesic, and a useful remedy against irritating cough. This would, in common consideration, designate it an herb. An appropriate herbal definition will distinguish food as sustenance from a substance consumed for psychological or physiological effect.

If we examine the botanical definition of an herb, we will see this definition lacks comprehensiveness as well: "A plant with a fleshy not a woody stem, which, after the plant has bloomed and set seed, dies down to the ground." This definition excludes plants such as barberry, cat's claw, and thyme. The barks of many plants are valuable medicinally and we, therefore, consider them herbs.

For the purposes of this book, we will formulate our own definition. An herb, sometimes known as a medicinal plant, is *a plant from which may be derived beneficial non-nutritive psychological or physiological effects, whether from ingestion, inhalation, or topical application.*

Today, tens of millions of people across the globe benefit from the active constituents in herbs. From health to culture to religion, plants play a part in our everyday life. Incense is often used as a spiritual symbol in churches and temples. With the development of Western medicine in the past century, herbalism declined in popularity, partially due to its association with archaic ritual and affiliation with magical beliefs. This is especially true in the United States. However, the past few decades have seen

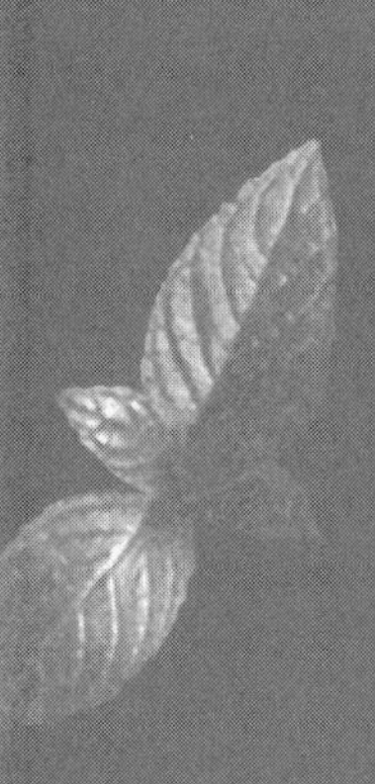

What is an Herb?

An herb is a plant from which may be derived beneficial non-nutritive psychological or physiological effects, whether from ingestion, inhalation, or topical application.

an upsurge of a naturalistic approach to health. Several reasons may account for this return to herbal practice:

- Scientific advancements have been able to verify and document the effects and active constituents of many herbs.
- The dangers and side effects of synthetic medications are better known.
- Certain bio-organisms have begun to resist particular synthetic medications.
- Herbalism affords the patient a greater independence and autonomy over traditional health care. Most medical professionals place patients in a passive role, and naturalistic medicine tends to encourage an active approach with collaborative treatment decisions, and patients' self-monitorization of results.

Alternative medicine offers a wider array of treatment options, which may fuel optimism and be emotionally attractive to the patient.

FROM PLANT TO PILL: SCIENTIFIC VERIFICATION OF HERBAL MEDICINE

Anyone questioning the value of herbal medicine need only note the powerful medications that were derived, then synthesized for modern use based upon the compounds discovered in plants.

Morphine — Morphine comes from the opium poppy (*Papaver rhoeas*).

Tubocurarine — The most powerful muscle relaxant in existence, tubocurarine is derived from the plant curare (*Chondrondendron tomestosum*). Aboriginal tribes in the Amazon used curare on arrow-points to paralyze animals when hunting.

Mexican Yam — Mexican yam (*Dioscorea* genus) yields diosgenin — an integral component in the synthesis of human sex hormones and the original chemical map for synthesized oral contraception.

Aspirin — Aspirin was derived from saliate discovered in 1827 and derived from the leaves of the meadowsweet plant (*Filipendula ulmaria*).

Anesthetics — Many come from the coca plant (*Erythroxylum coca*).

Dioxin — "The heart remedy" dioxin is derived from the common foxglove (*Digitalis purpurea*).

Quinine — An anti-malarial medication, quinine is derived from various species of cinchona or Peruvian bark.

Of course, there are many more examples of synthetic medication resulting from chemicals found in plant life. In fact, nearly 75 percent of our bioengineered medications have originated within the curative properties of plants. In the new millennium, the medical industry is closer than ever to integrating naturalistic medicine with the technological advantages of traditional heath care. Nearly 65 percent of medical schools in the United States offer some course work in alternative medicine, and this figure rises every year. "Alternative" medicine is becoming less an "alternative" and more a complement to medical treatment. In the way that diet, exercise, and stress management are recognized as crucial components in the treatment and prevention of ailments and the preservation of overall health, so too is herbal medicine becoming a routine corollary to traditional health avocations. Physicians in Europe and Asia routinely incorporate herbal remedies into their repertoire of prescriptions. The United States has been slower to embrace herbal remedies. This is, at least in part, due to the fact that the U.S. is significantly hampered by government restrictions that make it difficult for herbal substances to be commercially funded, tested, and distributed. In general, however, the trend in health care is definitely toward the recognition and incorporation of herbal medicine in standard medical practice.

This is where we are today. Let's take a look back at herbalism throughout the ages.

HERBAL HISTORY

From earliest times, man has benefited from the life-enhancing properties of plants. In the most primitive periods, man utilized plants as food, medicine, shelter, and tools with which to expand knowledge and survive. Plants also held an intricate connection to man's spiritual and magical beliefs. The oldest evidence of plants utilized by humans is a 60,000-year-old burial site from Mesopotamia (modern-day Iraq) that contained eight different herbs arranged about the corpse in a way to suggest the plants held spiritual as well as medicinal significance. Though historians believe the medicinal use of herbs precede this date, the oldest remaining physical evidence is significant. The most recent evidence tells us that this use of herbs predates the invention of the wheel by roughly 56,000 years. There can be no question as to the essential and fundamental connection of herbs and the physical and spiritual essence of human life.

The oldest written record of medicinal herbs comes much later on a 5,000-year-old Sumerian clay tablet that depicts several herbal remedies.

Egypt

In Ancient Egypt, medical practice combined herbalism, faith healing, and magic. One of the most significant records of Egyptian herbalism is a medicinal papyrus unearthed in the 19th century and translated by Georg Ebers. The Ebers Papyrus has been dated to c. 1552 BC and details remedies for more than one hundred ailments. The prescription for asthma, for example, was a crude vaporization method in which a precise herbal mixture was heated over a brick and inhaled. The papyrus also describes various com-

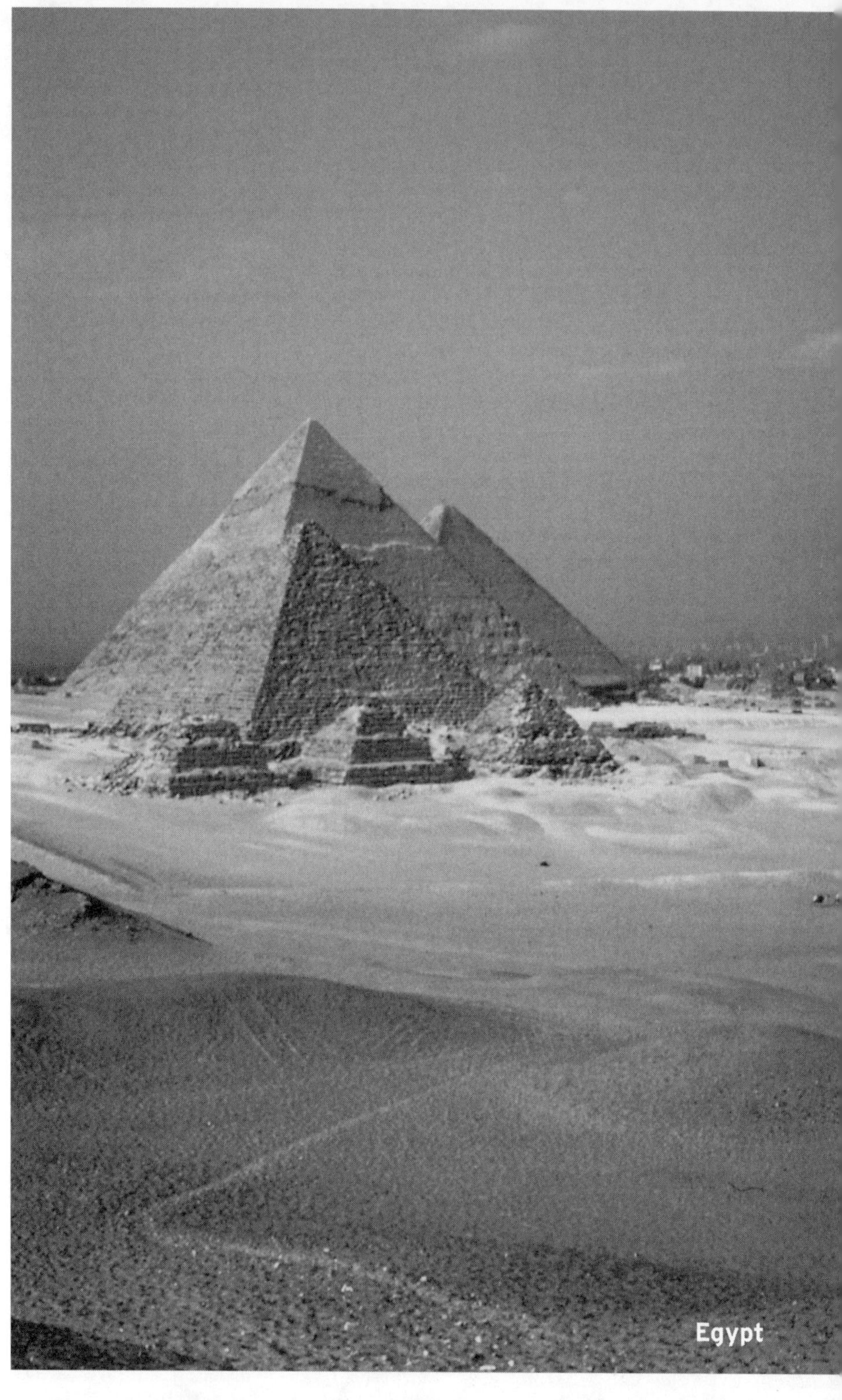

Egypt

mon ailments, protective incantations, and such valuable herbs as myrrh (*Commiphora molmol*), caraway (*Carum carvi*), and bayberry (*Myrica cerifera*). Many Egyptian treatments have since been proven to have sound medicinal properties. For example, honey was often used to heal wounds and today we understand honey's antibacterial properties.

India

The oral history of Indian culture and medicine were recorded in the Vedas, four books which detail, among other things, holistic medical practices, valuable herbs, cultural history, poetry, and folklore. This text was the first to assert that not a single plant on earth was without usefulness. "All the many herbs in which humans find remedy / Like Mothers gathered let them yield milk / Unto man, for freedom from harm." The Vedas, along with two later texts, (*Charaka Samhita* and *Sushruta Samhita*) laid the groundwork for the discipline of *Ayurveda*, which roughly translates to "the science of life, prevention, longevity". Ayurveda is an approach to wellness based on creating and maintaining an overall balance of health and well-being. This method advocates the internal and external use of herbs, attention to breathing and diet, and the practice of meditation and yoga. Ayurveda is not dissimilar to the herbal philosophy and technique of Ancient China, and is the basis for Indian herbal medicine even today.

Greece

By 400 BC, when herbal medicine had advanced in Greek, Roman and Egyptian cultures, the first real change in perspective was instigated by the Greek physician Hypocrites. Hypocrites treated ailments and their cures as physical, natural elements, rather than spiritual and supernatural. This was quite a contrast to the beliefs of the time. Aristotle had imbued plants with a sentient and ethereal essence, a soul. Illness was

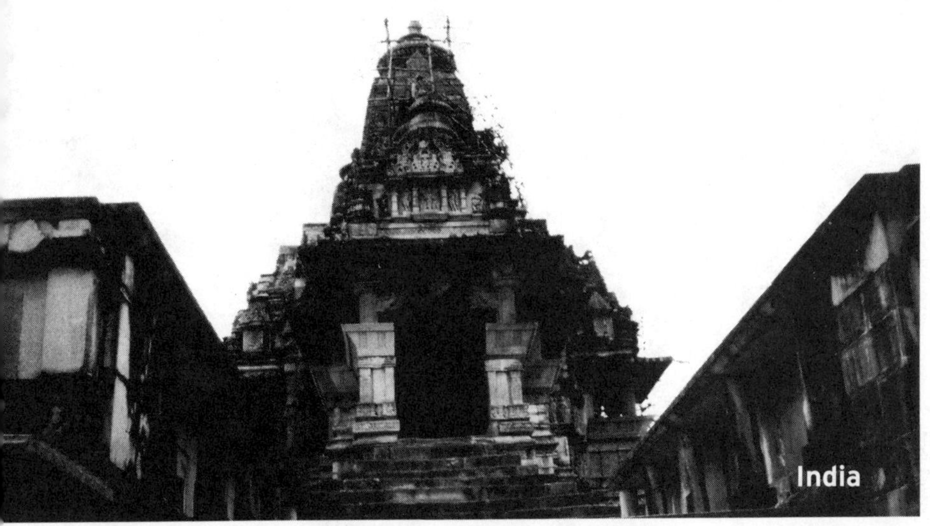
India

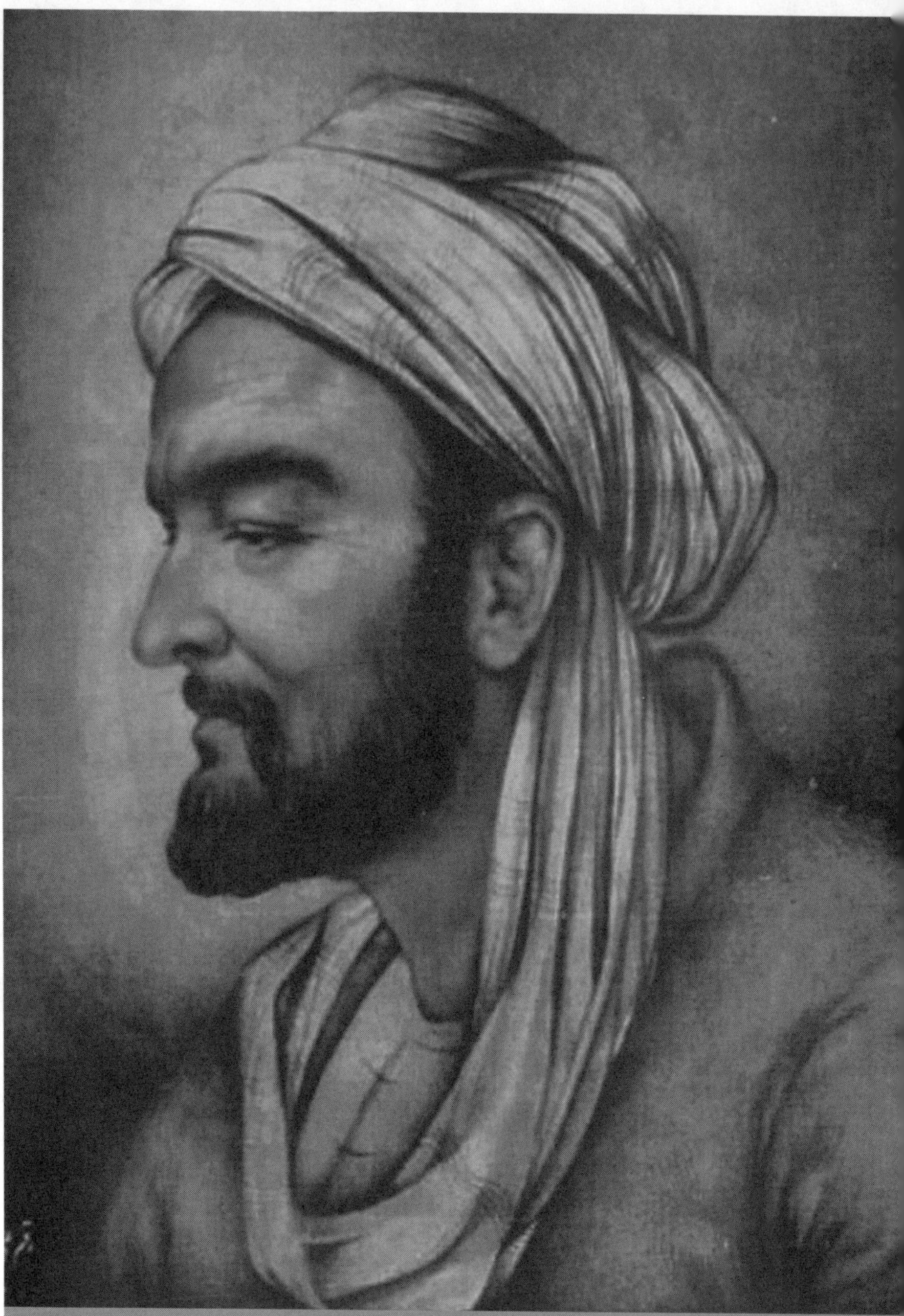

The Persian physician Avicenna (Ibn Sina), writer of 276 works covering medicine, natural history, physics, chemistry, mathematics, music, economics, morality and religion. Portrait courtesy of the National Library of Medicine.

often deemed more a possession of evil spirits, and treatments regarded as exorcism.

Even much later, Shamanistic practices involved the patient taking healing herbs while the shaman took hallucinogens in order ascend to the plane of evil spirits to fight them away from the afflicted body.

Hypocrites used direct observation, scrupulous records, and repeatable effects to document herbal uses. Hypocrites also advocated strengthening the body's natural defenses with air and proper diet as a way to prevent disease. This notion came to be the basis for what we know today as naturopathy.

China

Emperor Sheng Nung began his reign in 2,800 BC and became known to his people as the "father of agriculture", and later "the patron saint of herbology". He produced the first records of the actions of plants, often experimenting upon himself and, it is reputed, surviving numerous poisonings. Sheng Nung's work became the basis for one of the earliest herbals in existence: *The Divine Husbandman's Classic of The Materia Medica*, or *Sheng Nung Ben Cao Chien*. Often it is shortened to *Sheng Nung's Herbal*. Sheng Nung remains noted both for his astonishing accuracy in the details of 250 plants and 150 ailments and the development of the instrumental principal of Yin and Yang.

A few centuries later Huang Ti, infamously known as The Yellow Emperor, worked from Sheng Nung's herbal and further produced methods of diagnoses, extensive prescriptive herbs, and recorded the founding principals of Chinese Herbal Medicine. *The Yellow Emperor's Classic of Internal Medicine, Huang Ti Nei Ching*, or *Nei Ching*, for short. The *Nei Ching* was believed to have been written during Huang Ti's reign, around 2,500 BC,

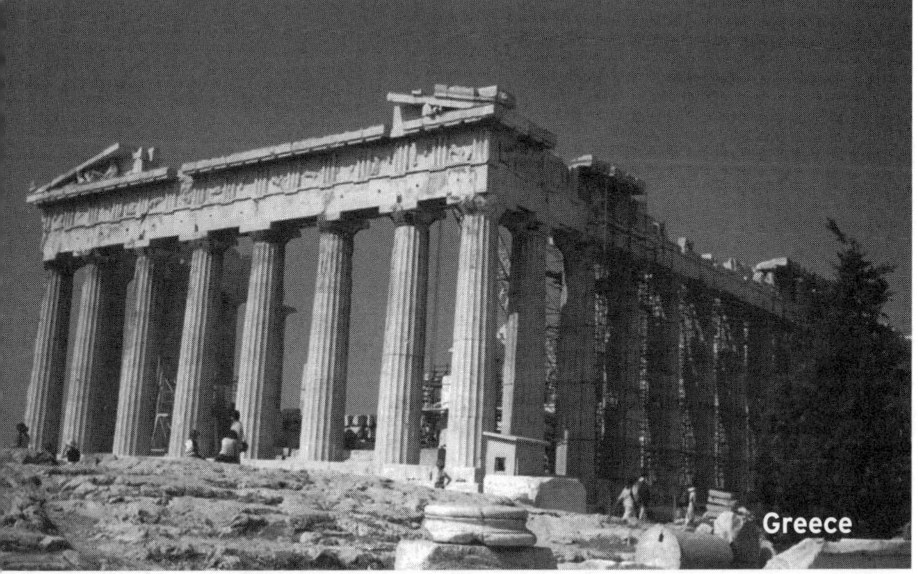

Greece

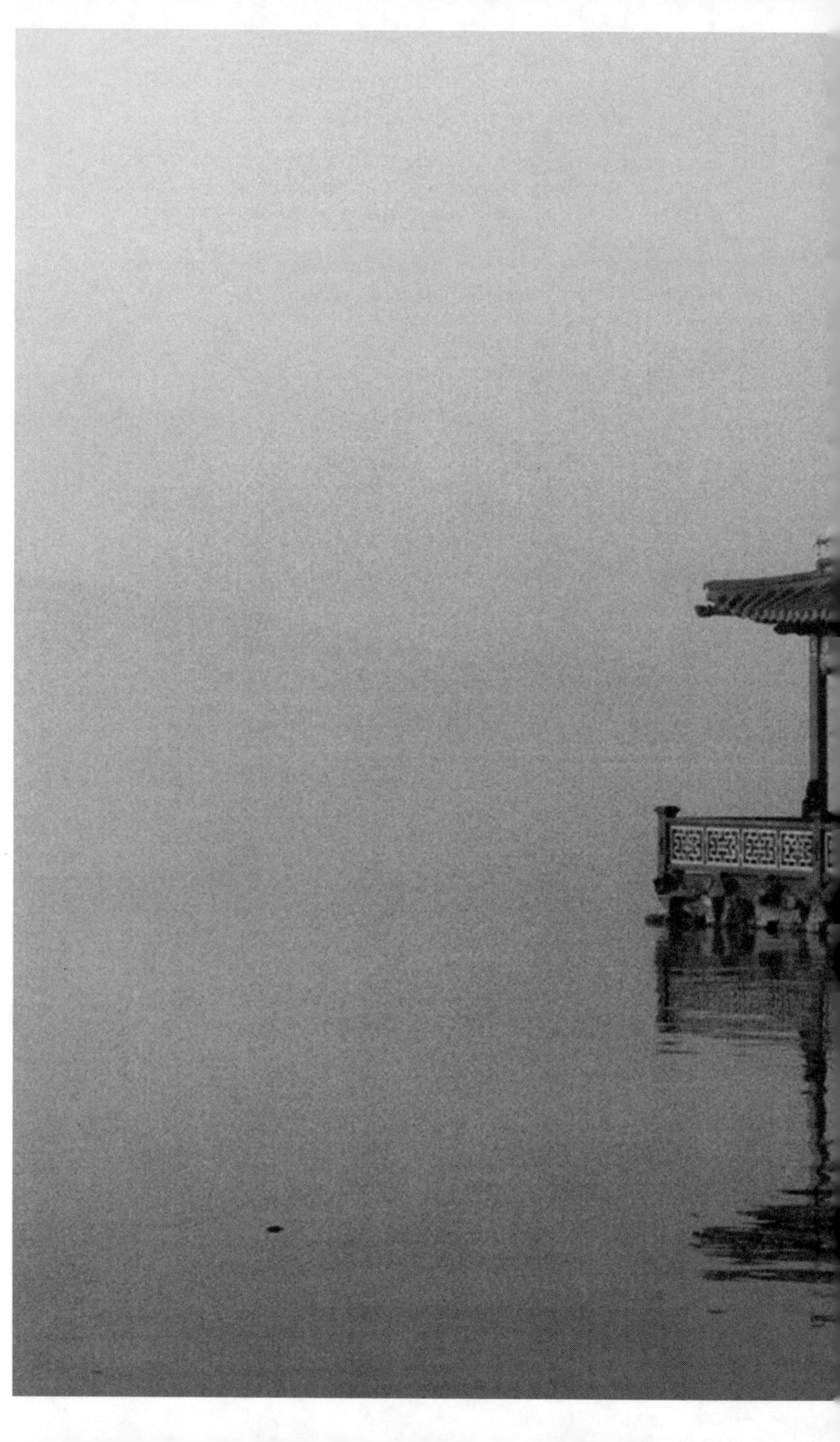

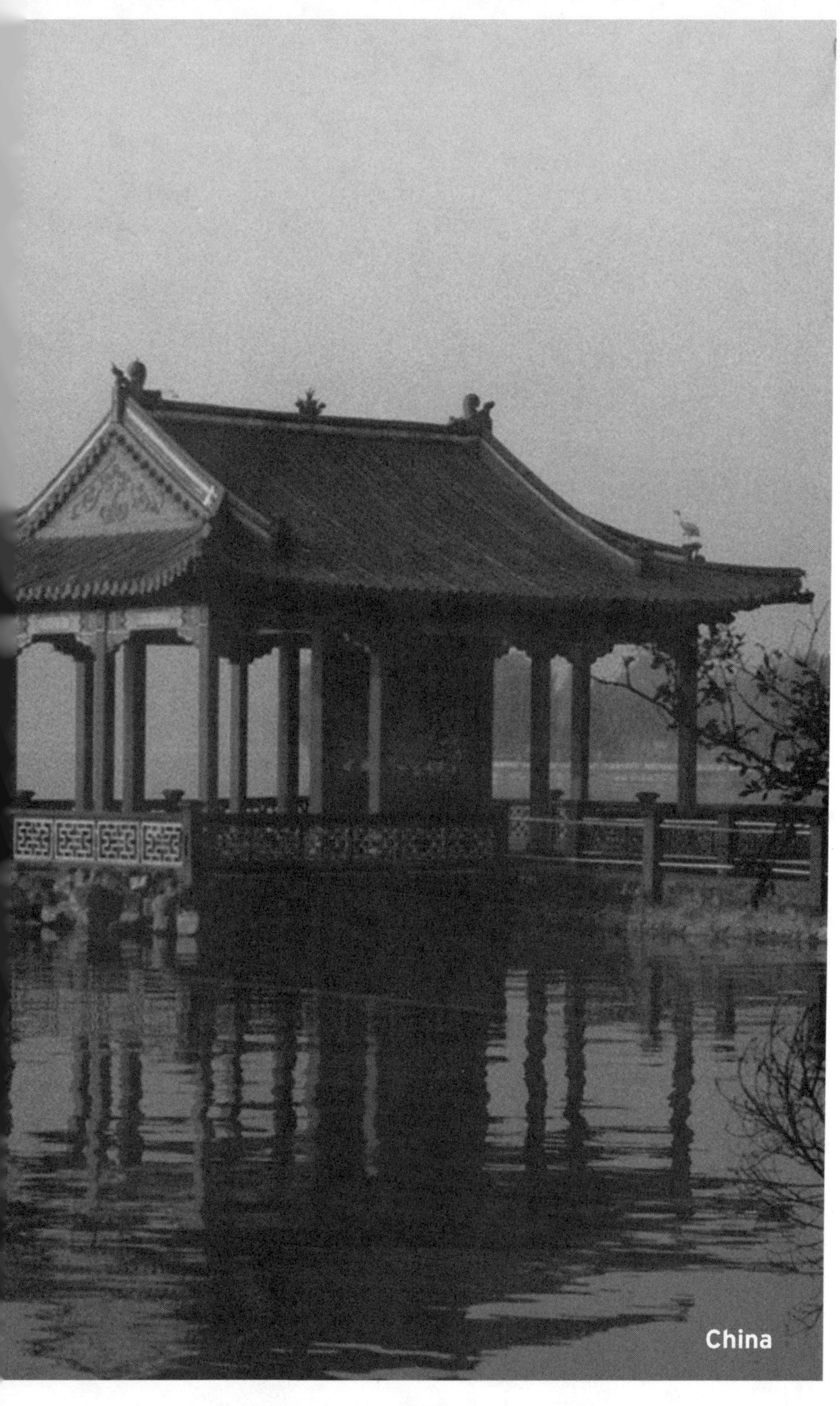

China

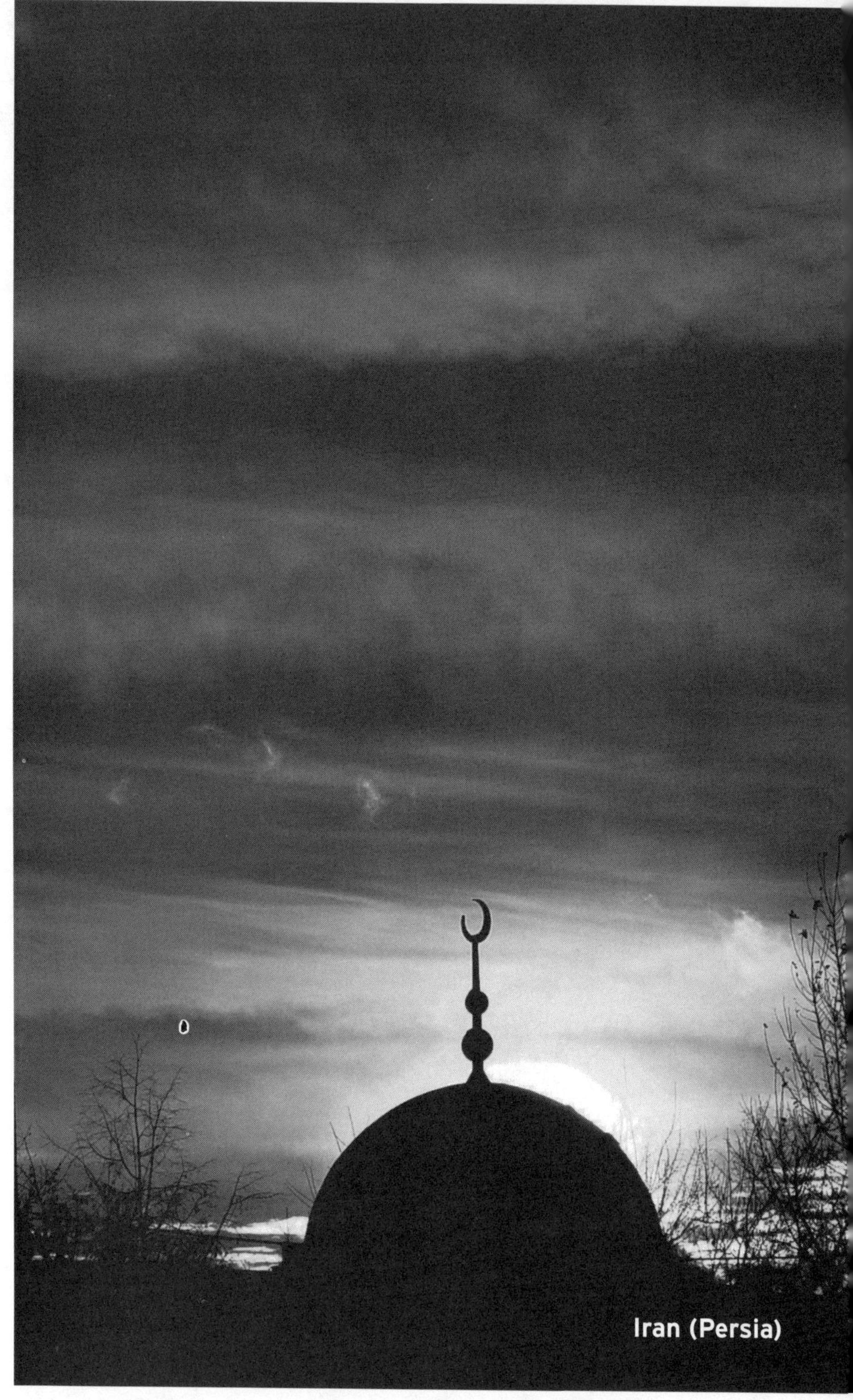

Iran (Persia)

though the earliest existing record of the herbal dates to 300 BC. This important text includes a thorough herbal pharmacopoeia, and extols the properties of the life-force energy *Qi*, the five phases of evolutionary change, and documented the principals of Yin and Yang, and the practice of acupuncture. Interestingly, this text was written in the form of a discussion between the Yellow Emperor and his minister, rather than as an instructional text.

Iran

During the Middle Ages, ancient Persians began to experiment with heating implements for their herbs. Herbs such as frankincense, benzoin and aloe wood were heated in bronze-cast braziers or atop flat warming-stones with a fire kindled beneath. These devices warmed a room and released healthful plant essences all at once.

Many of Persia's most profound contributions to the world of health and herbology, come from the research and writing of a single man.

Born in 980 AD, Ibn Sina (Hakim Abu Ali al-Husayn Abd Allah Ibn Sina), eventually known in the West as simply Avicenna, has been referred to as the most famous individual physician in the history of humanity. Referencing texts from memory, the Iranian physician wrote 276 books, which covered a vast range of topics including: medicine, natural history, physics, chemistry, mathematics, music, economics, morality and religion. His unprecedented work, *Kitab al-shifa'* or *The Book of Healing*, was extremely influential and is generally considered the largest volume ever produced by a single man. His second book sealed his infamy: *al-Qanun fi al-Tibb* or *The Canon of Medicine*. The *Encyclopædia Britannica* calls this work "the single most famous book in the history of medicine, in East or West." The *Canon* was comprised of five volumes that gathered and refined all of the medical knowledge in existence at the time.

Avicenna developed his theories of medicine through the related the doctrines of the natural sciences, and considered the evaluation of a "disease" incomplete until all components of a person had been included in the diagnosis.

Avicenna's works became the basis for most medieval schools of thought, especially that of the Franciscan monks, and through the ages has held vast influence on the development and practice of all medicine.

Through his teachings, Muslim civilizations made several very important contributions to medicine: developments in botany, pharmacy, and the founding of hospitals. Avicenna himself created a procedure of the distillation of floral oils and was the first to distill essence of rose. Centuries later, Avincenna's work inspired Samuel Hahnemann (1755–1843) to found homeopathy.

This gives you an idea of how ancient and intrinsic herbs are to human life. Let's examine how herbs are used today.

HERBS TODAY

There are more than 70,000 known species of plants in existence. The therapeutic effects of each plant and combinations of plants are virtually limitless. Advancements

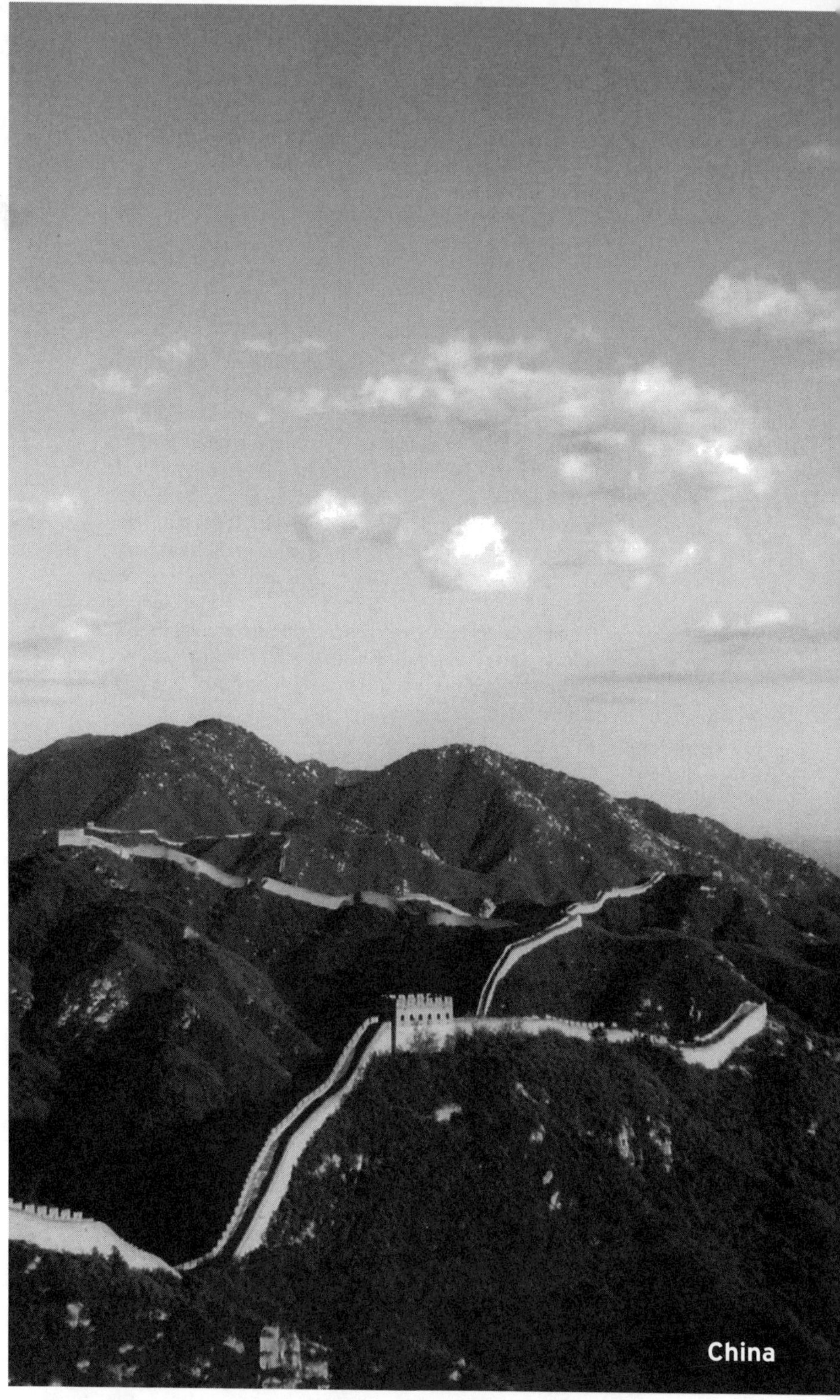
China

in science and individual and controlled experimentation lead to continual discovery of value and utility of plant life.

METHODS OF HERBAL DELIVERY

Several options are available for herbal use. Different herbs and different ailments will lend themselves to various modes of delivery. Bronchial ailments, for example, do well with inhaled vapors, while cuts and burns are best aided by external application. Choice of delivery mode depends upon circumstance and individual preference.

Ingestion

Infusion — Infusions are basically brewing an herb into a tea. Dried or fresh herbs may be used, however dried herbs require only ⅓ of the recommended dose for a fresh herb, because fresh herbs hold a high water content. Simply mix the herbs in a teapot with boiling water, then strain before consuming. Infusions work best with leaves, flowers, and green stems. Heavier material such as root or bark should be ground to power before attempting to infuse. Be careful that your herb doesn't have highly volatile oil or its constituents may break down under the heat of boiling water. Cold infusions may be used in this case.

Decoction — A decoction is simply a more strenuous method of infusion. Decoctions work best with woody substances such as, bark, woody stem, root, or seeds. Cover herbs with cold water in a saucepan and bring to a boil. Simmer the herbs for 20 – 30 minutes until liquid is reduced by roughly one third. Then strain the liquid and store in a cool area.

Tincture — Tinctures extract the essence of an herb through absorption in alcohol, usually vodka or rum. (Never use industrial, methyl, or rubbing alcohol.) Non-alcoholic tinctures may be made with vinegar or glycerol. Tinctures produce a strong elixir and if stored properly will last up to two years. However, they require a somewhat lengthy preparation, and are best made with the aid of a wine press.

Capsules and Powder — Powered herbs may be taken in capsule form, sprinkled over food or stirred into a beverage. The powdered form of an herb is also useful as a base for a poultice or ointment.

Syrup — Adding honey or sugar to an infusion or decoction will act as a preservative and taste enhancer, and is soothing for some ailments including sore throat or irritating cough. The mixture should be simmered for 15-30 minutes and stored in a sealable dark glass container.

Caution!

If you are pregnant:

- Avoid all medications including herbs for the first three months of pregnancy, unless otherwise directed by a medical professional.
- Avoid herbal tinctures for the entire term.
- Avoid rue, cat's claw, feverfew, motherwort, sage, and thyme for the entire term.

If you are taking prescription medication:

- Consult a physician before embarking on an herbal regime.

Store-bought essential oils should never be directly ingested.

External Application

Note: Topically applied herbs may cause skin irritation. Test for a short amount of time before prolonged external use of an herb.

Ointment — Ointments mix an oil or fat substance with an herb for a spreadable topical agent. Petroleum jelly or wax is often used. Ointments can be made to different consistencies depending on their application. For instance, a lip balm would be very thick while a burn ointment would be a bit thinner. Ointments require a lengthy preparation.

Cream — A cream is an ointment with a higher amount of water. Creams will blend with the skin and may have a cooling and soothing effect. Like ointments, creams require proper time and equipment.

Poultice — A poultice is a mixture of herbs, undiluted, and applied to the skin with a cloth or bandage. Poultices may be used to ease nerve, joint or muscle pain, and to heal open wounds or sores.

Inhalation

Aroma vaporizers release steam and the user enjoys the restorative or stimulating properties of the scent. This method is now empowered with the concentrated and precise abilities of digital vaporization technology. With this technology, inhalation is a quick, economical, and effective way to receive the benefits of your favorite herb. As discussed in Chapter 1, herbs are heated to their vaporization point, and the essential oils are released in a pure cloud of vapor, which is inhaled.

Vaporization offers certain benefits over traditional herbal delivery systems.

Herbs to Avoid During Pregnancy

Barberry
Bearberry
Black Cohost
Black Walnut Hulls
Blueberry
Blue Cohosh
Catnip
Caparral
Dong Quai
Ephedra
Goldenseal
Juniper Berry

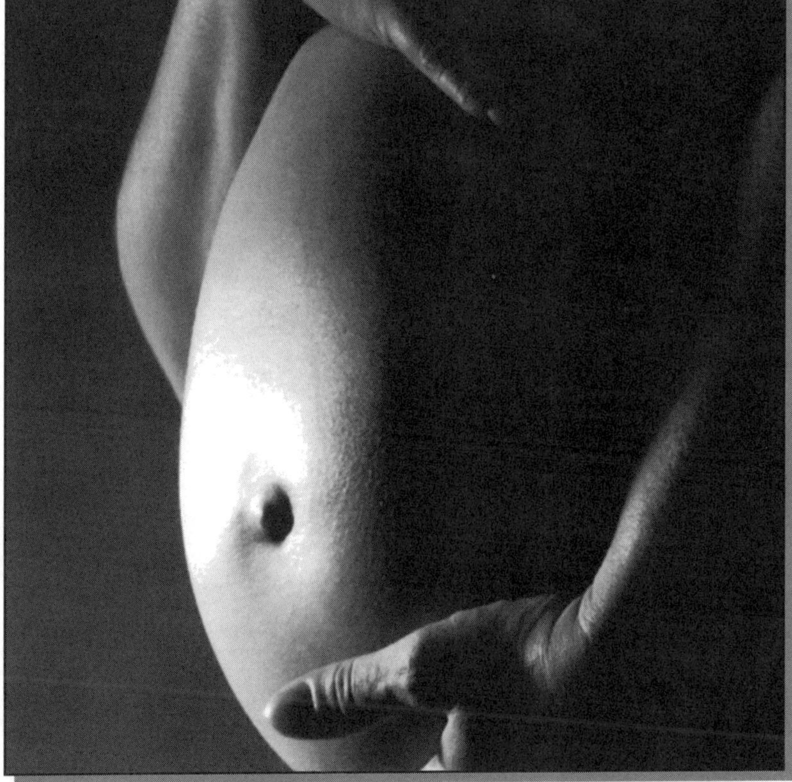

• Herbs are absorbed from the lungs directly into the bloodstream. Therefore the effects of many herbs are near immediate. This is useful in controlling the dose. Ingested herbs have a delay-of-effect and are taken in a packaged dose. Often the user will ingest more herb than necessary for the desired effect. Although side effects in herbal remedies are uncommon, this does result in a waste of herbal material.
• Purity — when taken orally, the active constituents of an herb are broken down by digestive acids and reach the bloodstream in an impure form.
• With vaporization, the user receives the pure active elements.

Use Herbs Wisely

Herbal medicines are generally safe and produce few side effects. Be sure to use only the part of the plant indicated and consult a professional before determining herbal medicine as your primary form of self-treatment. Be aware that, although it's rare, herbs may contraindicate synthetic medication. There are cases where the guidance of a medical professional is clearly the safest course of action. If you suffer from a life-threatening disease, have severe allergic reactions, or see no improvement in symptoms for two or more weeks, seek professional advice.

Each individual has his or her own unique reaction to an herb. Experiment with herb combinations, recommended dosage, and method of delivery. Keep track of your responses and use this information to determine the herbal conditions right for you. For total health and well being, supplement your herbal treatment with proper diet, exercise, and stress-management.

Body Tonics: Tonics are herbs that enhance the vitality and overall strength of the body, or a particular body system. They typically increase circulation, fortify tissue, and nourish and tone muscle and organs. Tonics may be taken as a preventive aid, or in response to a specific malady.

Cardiovascular System: Heart tonics usually include circulatory stimulants and diaphoretics. They may stimulate or slow heart rate and regulate and strengthen pulse. *Garlic, Hawthorn, Buckwheat, Arjuna, Broom, Squill. Cayenne, Crampbark*

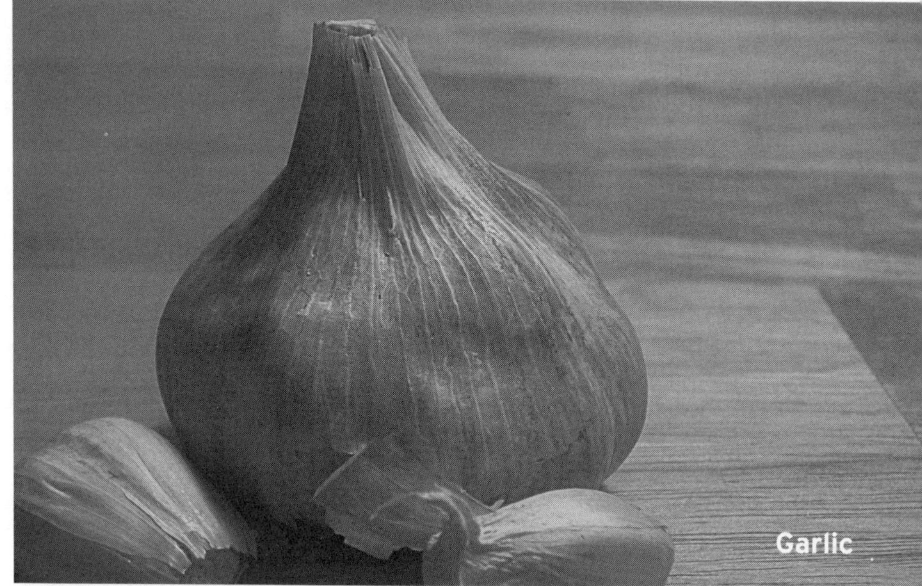
Garlic

Nervous System: Nervous tonics work to restore balance, or homeostasis, in the nervous system and between the nervous system and the rest of the body. They may suppress or increase nervous activity, improve nerve cell reaction, and restore the system as a whole. *Rosemary, Skullcap, Saint-John's-Wort, Oats*

Immune System: Immune System tonics strengthen white blood cells and ready the body to fight viruses, bacteria, or parasites. *Echinacea, Lapacho, Garlic, Barberry*

Respiratory System: Respiratory tonics increase blood flow and oxygenation of the cells throughout the body. They clarify and tone the lungs, break down respiratory catarrhal and ensure proper airflow. *Elecampane, Colt's Foot, Marshmallow, Garlic*

Digestive System: Bitter tonics soothe an uneasy stomach and facilitate the digestion process. They are often antiseptics, bitters, carminatives, and cholagogues. *Agrimony, Dandelion Root, Gentian*

Skin: Skin tonics often include antiseptics, astringents, emollients, and vulnerary herbs, to tone, disinfect, remove sub-dermal waste, and heal wounds. *Burdock, Cleavers, Nettles, Comfrey*

Urinary System: Urinary tonics improve circulation, tone the liver, and aid in the removal of toxins from the body. Tonics for the urinary system are frequently diuretics, antiseptics, bitters, and hepatics. *Milk Thistle, Horsetail, Corn Silk*

Musculoskeletal System: These tonics help strengthen bone and connective tissue. They may relieve joint pain, nerve pain, reduce swelling, or ease cramped muscles.

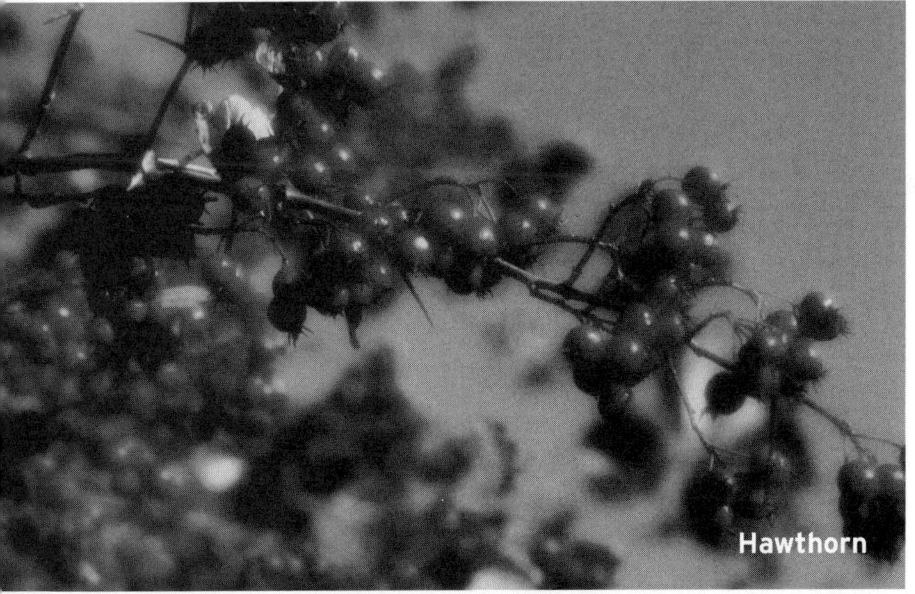
Hawthorn

Analgesics and antispasmodics are common in a musculoskeletal tonic. *Passionflower, Chamomile, Saint-John's-Wort, Valerian*

ANTI-AGING HERBS

The youth-preserving properties of these herbs compliment a healthy lifestyle of balanced diet, positive outlook and regular activity.

Celery Seed *Apium graveolens*
Studies have shown celery seed may lower high blood pressure and is filled with anti-inflammatory agents that may alleviate symptoms of gout and arthritis.

Echinacea ***Echinacea*, Various Species**
Echinacea is a great immune-system enhancer.

Evening Primrose *Oenathera biennis*
This herb is filled with gamma-linolenic acid (GLA), a substance believed to guard against heart disease. Evening primrose also helps prevent menstrual cramps.

Garlic *Allium sativum*
A "veritable wonder herb". Garlic is a potent antimicrobial which helps defeat a wide range of viruses, bacteria, and fungi. It also lowers blood pressure and cholesterol, and inhibits the formation of blood clots, which may trigger arterial disease, aneurysm, or stroke. Clinical research suggests that garlic helps to slow age-related memory-loss in animals.

Gingko *Gingko biloba*
Gingko improves blood flow, enhances memory, and holds the potential to prevent stroke and Alzheimer's disease.

Hawthorn *Crataegus monogyna*
Hawthorn normalizes heart function.

Horse Chestnut *Aesculus hippocastanum*
Horse chestnut is an excellent remedy for varicose veins. *Note*: Never take fresh horse chestnut internally; it is poisonous. Commercial preparations are detoxified.

Kava Kava *Piper methysticum*
Kava kava is a stress reliever. It helps prevent stress-related aliments which are a major contributor to aging. There has been recent controversy over the safety of kava kava, particularly in relation of liver disease. Many herbalists, who have been safely using and prescribing kava kava for decades, suspect that this concern will soon prove to be without merit.

Herbs to Avoid

The following herbs can potentially be toxic and should be used cautiously and in many cases under the care of a trained practitioner:

Apple (Balsam), *Momordica balsamina*
Apple (Bitter), *Citrullus colocynthis*
American mistletoe
Baneberry, Actaea spicata
Belladonna (Deadly Nightshade), *Atropa belladonna*
Bloodroot, *Sanguinaria candensis*
Bryony, Black, *Tamus communis*
Bryony, European, *Bryonia alba*
Bryony, White, *Bryonia dioica*
Cabbage Tree, *Andira inermis*
Calabar Bean, *Physostigma venenosum*
Calotropis, *Physostigma venenosum*
Cherry Laurel, *Prunus laurocerasus*
Chaparral, *Larrea tridentata*
Clematis, *Clematis recta*
Coca, Bolivian, *Erythroxylon coca*
Cocculus, Indicus, *Anamirta paniculata*
Dropwort / Hemlock Water, *Oenanthe crocata*
Foxglove, *Digitalis purpurea*
Gelsemium, *Gelsemium nitidum*
Hellebore, Black, *Helleborus niger*
Hellebore, False, *Adonis autumnalis*
Hellebore, Green, *Veratrum viride*
Hellebore, White, *Veratrum album*
Hemlock, *Conium maculatum*
Hemlock, Water, *Cicuta virosa*
Ignatius Beans, *Strychnos ignatii*
Ivy, Poison, *Rhus toxicodendron*
Laburnum, *Cytisus laburnam*
Laurel, Mountain, *Kalmia latifolia*
Madagascar Periwinkle, *Vinca rosea*
Mandrake (aerial parts), *Mandragora officinarum*
Mescal Buttons, *Anhalonium lewinii*
Nightshade, Black, *Solanum nigrum*
Nux Vomica, *Strychnos Nux-vomica*
Paris, herb, *Paris quadrifolia*
Pokeweed, *Phytolacca decandra*
Thornapple, *Datura stramonium*
Wake Robin, American, *Arum triphyllum*
Yew, *Taxus baccata*

Milk Thistle *Silybum marianum*
This is the best herb for your liver. Milk thistle safeguards against cirrhosis and hepatitis. New evidence reveals milk thistle's ability to prevent cancer, type 2 diabetes, and syndrome X.

Saint-John's-Wort *Hypericum perforatum*
This herb aids the function of the immune system and may alleviate mild to moderate depression.

Saw Palmetto *Serenoar repens*
Many use this herb to treat prostate problems. Be sure to see doctor for proper diagnosis.

Turmeric *Curcuma longa*
Turmeric relieves general aches and pains. Its anti-inflammatory properties make it helpful with arthritis, bursitis, and tendonitis.

American and Asian Ginseng *Panax quinquefolius* **and** *Panax ginseng*
Ginseng translates to "wonder of the world", though in China and Korea you may hear ginseng referred to as "The Fountain of Youth". This herb has proven an extremely effective tonic for the elderly. It can tone muscles and skin, improve appetite and digestion, and restore sexual energies. Andrew Weil MD highly recommends ginseng to patients "weakened by old age or chronic illness".

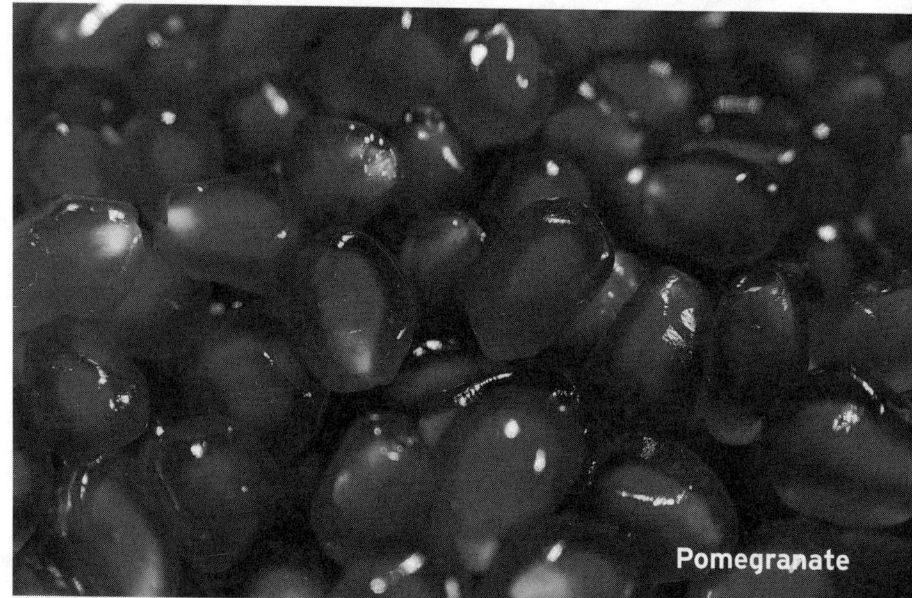
Pomegranate

Gotu Kola *Centella asiatica*
Gotu kola has been long valued in Ayurvedi medicine for its power to improve memory and extend longevity.

Peppermint *Mentha poperita*
Peppermint is the perfect remedy for gastro-intestinal discomfort. It is also filled with anti-oxidants, which help prevent age-related disease.

Purslane *Portulaca oleracea*
Purslane is one of the most nutritious herbs in existence. It provides a tremendous amount of potassium, and is rich in omega-3 fatty acids. These acids are an excellent protective agent for the heart. Purslane is also a strong diuretic; it aids in the management of high blood pressure, and studies indicate purslane may regulate blood sugar and manage diabetes.

Horsetail *Equisetum arvense*
Horsetail is an outstanding source of silicon, which can help strengthen bones and prevent fractures and breaking.

WOMEN'S HEALTH

These herbs strengthen bones, regulate menstruation, and provide nutrients specific to the female body.

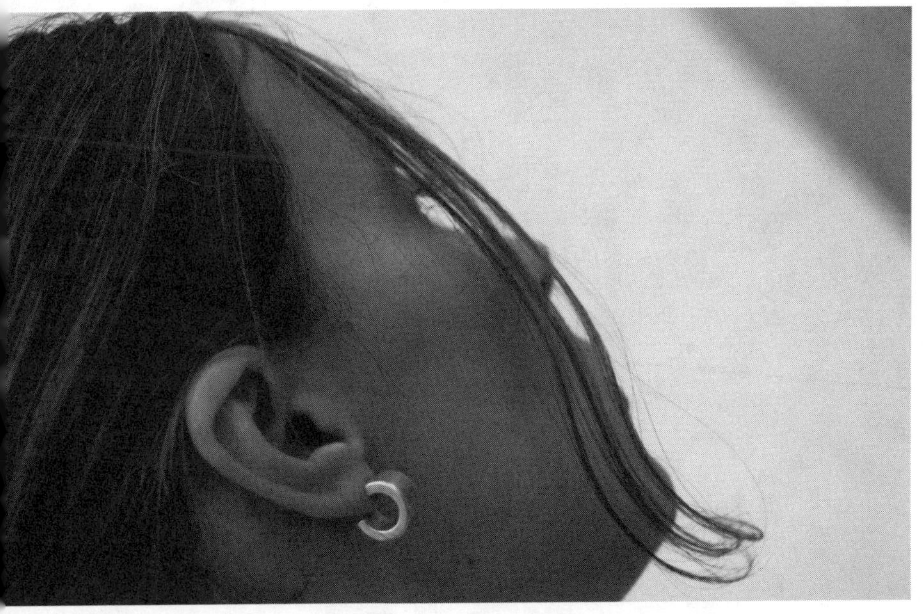

The Female Reproductive System:
Black Horehound *Ballota nigra*
Chaste Tree *Vitex agnus-castus*
Dong Quai *Angelica sinensis*
Squaw Vine *Mitchella repens*
Blue Cohosh *Cimicifuga racemosa*
Goldenseal *Hydratis canadenis*
Sage *Salvia officinalis*

Menstrual Pain:
Black Haw *Viburnum prunifolium*
Native Americans and colonial women used Black Haw to relieve menstrual pain. This herb contains four different compounds which help to relax the uterus.
Cramp Bark *Viburnum opulus*
Raspberry *Rubus idaeus*
American Partridgeberry *Mitchella repens*
Black Cohosh *Cimicifuga racemosa*
Wild Yam *Dioscorea villosa*
Combo: Equal parts Wild Yam, Black Haw, Cramp Bark — Flavored with Caraway seeds

Pre-Menstrual Syndrome:
Dong Quai *Angelica sinensis*
Damiani *Turnera aphrodisiaca*

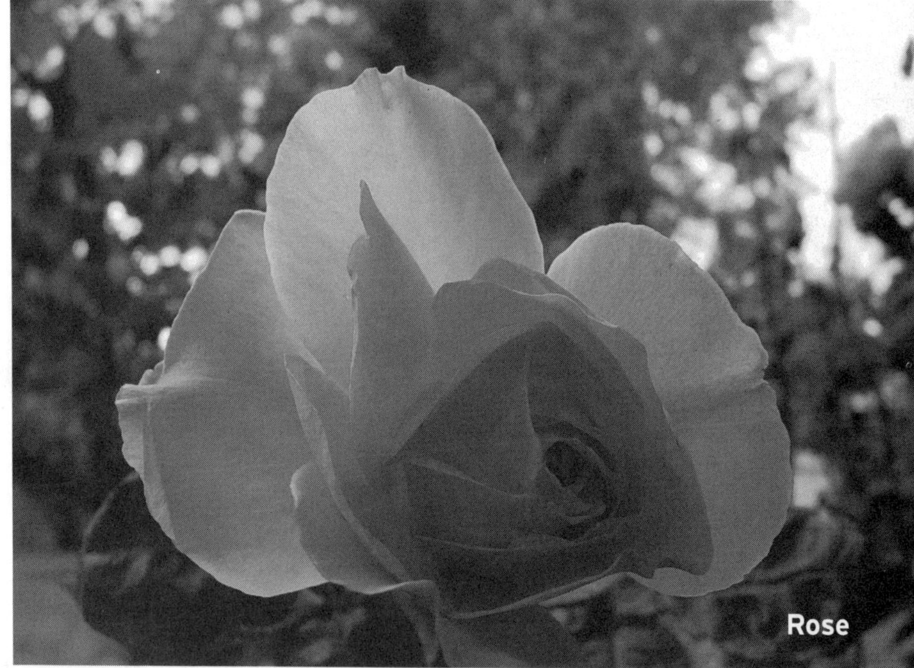
Rose

Ying Ywanghuo *Epimedium, VS*
Anise *Pimpinella anisum*
Fennel *Foeniculum vulgare*
Fenugreek *Trigonella foenum-graecum*
Ginger *Zingiber officinale*
Asian Ginseng *Panax ginseng*
Wild Yam *Dioscorea villosa*

Menopause:
Black Cohosh *Cimicifuga racemosa*
Licorice *Glycyrrhiza glabra*
Chasteberry *Vitex agnus-castus*
Pomegranate *Punica granatum (for hot flashes)*
Red Clover *Trifolium pratense*
Evening Primrose *Cenothera biennis*
Fenugreek
Kudzu

Breast Enlargement:
Fenugreek
For centuries this herb has been a folk remedy for enhancing breast size and although no studies have been conducted, modern testimonials give good evidence to its efficacy. Fenugreek seeds contain diosgenin, which is a chemical compound often used to synthesize a form of the female sex hormone estrogen.
Fennel
This is another estrogen producing herb which has been used for centuries to promote the flow of milk in nursing mothers. In a non-pregnant female, it has the same effect as fenugreek.
Saw Palmetto
Best known for its ability to shrink an enlarged prostate in men, saw palmetto has also been applied for breast enlargement purposes.

MEN'S HEALTH

Reproduction and Sexual Function:
Gingko *Gingko biloba*
Asian Ginseng *Panax ginseng*
Yohimbe *Pausinystalia yohimbe ("Erection Enhancer")*
Quebracho *Aspidosperma quebracho-blanco*
Wild Oates *Avena sativa*
Yinyanghuo *Epimedium, VS*
Cocoa cream *Theobroma cacao*
Garlic *Allium sativa*
Muira Puama *Ptychopetalum olacoides*

Oxeye *Mucuna, VS*
Withania *Withania somnifera*
Saw Palmetto *Sabal serrulata*

Baldness:
Saw Palmetto
Blocks the formation of DHT which is known to kill hair follicles.
Licorice
Prevents conversion of testosterone to DHT.
Rosemary
Use direct application in a poultice or compress.
Horsetail
Contains minerals selenium and silicon which "help promote circulation to the scalp".
Safflower *Carthamus tinctorius*
Chinese believe this herb open blood vessels in the scalp thereby aiding the flow of nutrients to the hair follicles.
Stinging Nettle
Strongly advocated by the imminent German herbalist Rudolf Fritz Weiss, MD.

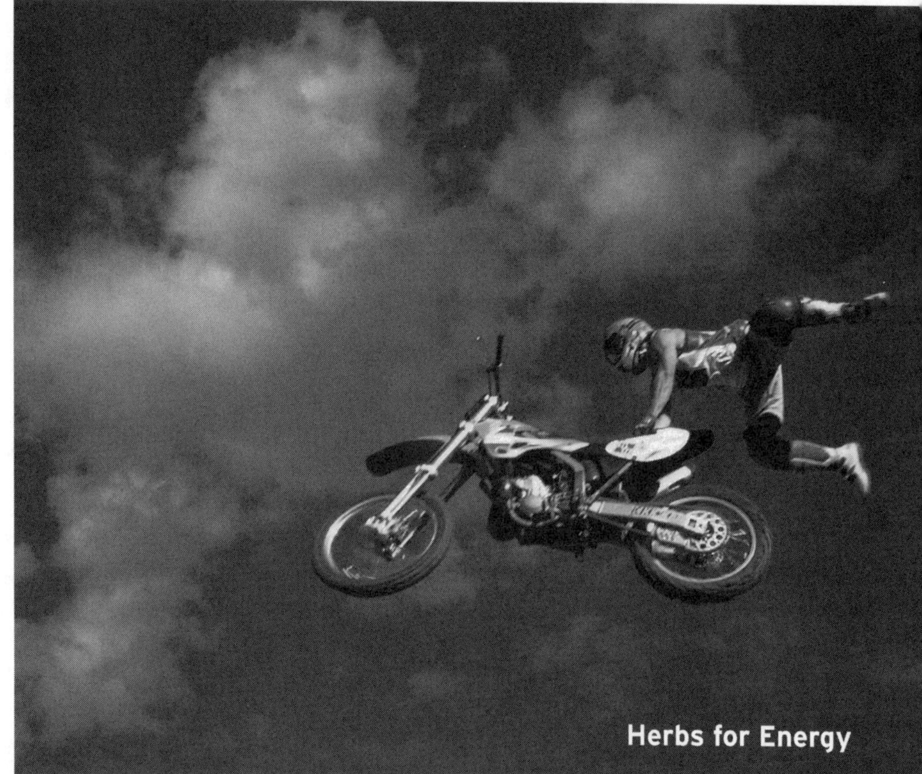

HERBS FOR ENERGY AND MENTAL ACUITY

These herbs contain high levels of cineole, a substance which sharpens mental ability, increases circulation, and improves baseline vitality. Cineole provides a subtler and long-lasting lift than more robust stimulants such as caffeine.

Cardamom *Elettaria cardamomum*
Eucalyptus *Eucalyptus globulus*
Spearmint *Mentha viridis*
Rosemary *Rosmarinus officinalis*
Ginger *Allium sativum*
Nutmeg *Myristica fragrans*
Peppermint *Mentha piperita*
Yarrow *Achillea millefolium*

Stress Busters:
(Herbs to calm anxiety and soothe mild depression)
Valerian *Valeriana Officinalis*
Saint-John's-Wort *Hypericum perforatum*
Hop *Humulus lupulus*
Passionflower *Passiflora incarnata*
Chamomile *Anthemis nobilis*
Bergamot *Monarda didyma*
Lavender *Lavandula, VS relaxant,*
Rose *Rosa gallica*
Especially good for post-natal malaise.
Sandalwood *Santalum album*
Cranesbill Root *Geranium maculatum*
Recommended in small quantities.
Ylang Ylang *Cananga odorata*
Frankincense *Boswellia thurifera*
Calms the body and deepens breathing, great for meditation.
Bitter Orange *Citrus aurantium*
Calms the body, encourages sleep.

OTHER USES FOR HERBS

Arthritis:
Black Cohosh
Bogbean
Celery Seed
Prickly Ash
Wild Yam

Asthma:
Elecampane
Epherdra
Lobelia
Wild Cherry

High Blood Pressure:
Hawthorn
Lime Blossom
Yarrow

Bronchitis:
Bloodroot
Colt's Foot
Echinacea
Elecampane
Comfrey
Fenugreek
White horehound

Cholesterol:
Ginger
Hawthorn
Mukul
Turmeric

Cold and Flu:
Angelica
Boneset
Cayenne
Echinacea
Elder
Garlic
Ginger
Goldenseal
Hyssop
Peppermint
Yarrow

Eczema and Psoriasis:
Blue Flag
Burdock
Chickweed
Cleavers
Figwort
Goldenseal

Gall-Bladder Ailments:
Balmony
Blackroot
Dandelion
Fringe Tree
Milk Thistle
Wild Yam

Headache:
Betony
Feverfew
Rosemary
Skullcap

Infection:
Cleavers
Echinacea
Garlic
Goldenseal
Myrrh

Nausea:
Black Horehound
Chamomile
Meadowsweet
Peppermint

Wounds:
Comfrey
Elder
Goldenseal
Marigold
Saint-John's-Wort

GLOSSARY OF THERAPEUTIC ACTIONS

Alternative
Once know as "blood cleansers" alternatives are herbs that affect the body gradually and whose initial effect may go unnoticed. These herbs are often brewed in teas. and their benefits build over time as they work to remove toxins, restore vitality and strengthen overall bodily function. Examples: Burdock, Echinacea, Goldenseal

Analgesic / Anodyne
Painkillers. An analgesic is a stronger remedy for pain, however an anodyne may contribute an anesthetic effect as well and can be used to induce an unconscious state. Examples: Passionflower, Red Poppy, Saint-John's-Wort

Anthelmintic (Vermicide / Vermifuge)
These herbs will kill or destroy intestinal worms. Some anthelmintic herbs may be toxic in high dosage. Examples: Garlic, Wormwood, Rue

Anti-Bilious
These herbs remove excess bile from the body and may be useful in treating jaundice or biliary conditions. Examples: Barberry, Dandelion, Goldenseal

Antibiotic
Antibiotics destroy or inhibit the growth of bacteria, viruses, and other microorganisms in the body. Examples: Echinacea, Goldenseal, Myrrh

Anti-Catarrhal
Anti-catarrhals counteract the formation and inflammation of mucus, especially in the nose and throat. Examples: Garlic, Goldenrod, Hyssop

Anti-Emetic
Anti-emetic herbs suppress or prevent nausea and vomiting. Examples: Black Horehound, Meadowsweet, Fennel

Anti-Hydrotic
Produces an inhibitory action on the secretion of sweat. Examples: Sage, Lavender, Zizyphus

Anti-Inflammatory
These herbs reduce inflammation. Examples: Chamomile, Cat's Claw, Saint-John's-Wort

Anti-Lithic
Anti-lithics dissolve and prevention further formation of urinary or biliary stones. Examples: Corn Silk, Gravel Root, Hydrangea

Anti-Microbial
These herbs destroy or inhibit the growth of destructive microorganisms. Examples: Clove, Echinacea, Wormwood

Anti-Pyretic (Febrifuge)
Anti-pyretics are "cooling" herbs used in fever reduction Examples: Alfalfa, Skullcap, Yarrow

Antiseptic
These herbs fight infection by suppressing and preventing the growth of microbes and bacteria. Examples: Burdock, Goldenseal, Sage

Anti-Spasmodic
Anti-spasmodic herbs prevent or ease muscle spasms and cramps. Examples: Lobelia, Skullcap, Valerian

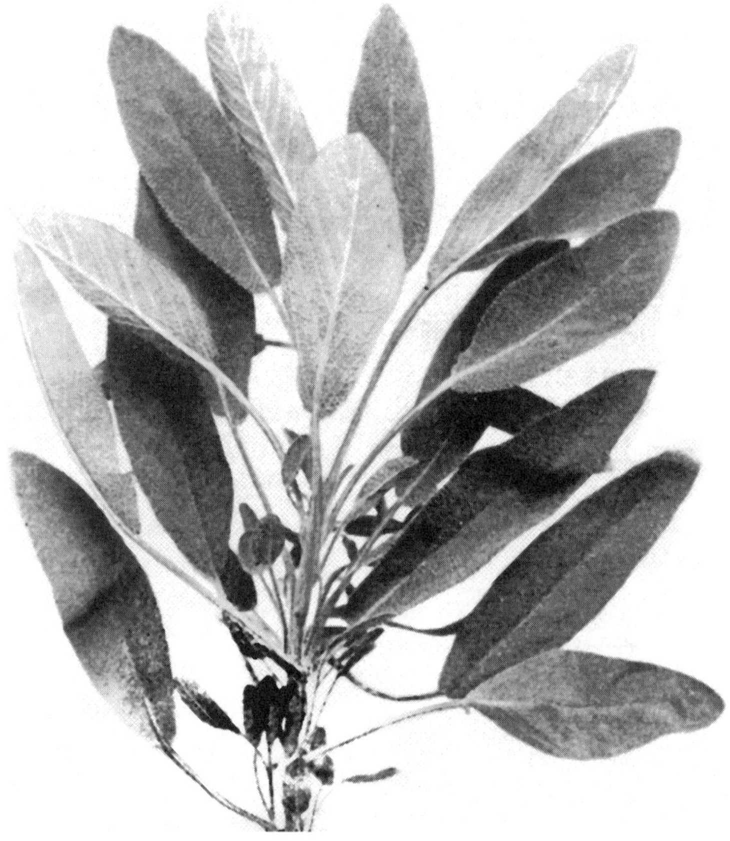

Aromatic
Aromatic herbs emit a strong, pleasant fragrance that often has the effect of stimulating and aiding the digestive process. Aromatics may be mixed with other herbs and medicines to improve taste and aroma. Examples: Angelica, Chamomile, Peppermint

Astringent
An astringent contracts tissues to reduce secretions. Astringents work both internally and externally. Examples: Agrimony, Bayberry, Yarrow

Antioxidant
Herbs with antioxidant actions prevent or delay the damaging oxidization of the body's cells. Examples: Gingko, Licorice, Turmeric

Bitter
The bitter flavor of these herbs ranges from mild to distinctly unpleasant. Through the taste buds, bitters stimulate the digestive system, and aid gastric function. Examples: Dandelion, Gentian, Hops

Carminative
The rich volatile oils of carminatives stimulate digestion and promote the expulsion of excess gas. Examples: Aniseed, Caraway, Peppermint

Cholagogue
These herbs aid with problems of the gall-bladder by stimulating its secretion of bile. They may also act as an all-natural laxative. Examples: Dandelion, Fringe Tree, Wild Yam

Cytostatic
Inhibiting or suppressing cellular growth and multiplication. Examples: Cat's Claw, Mandrake Root

Demulcent
These soothing substances heal and protect inflamed tissue, especially of the digestive tract, and reduce irritation in the urinary and respiratory systems. Examples: Comfrey, Corn Silk, Slippery Elm

Diaphoretic
Diaphoretic herbs induce perspiration to cool fever and stimulate the release of toxins from the body. Examples: Elder, Ginger, Yarrow

Diuretic
Diuretics stimulate urination to relieve bloating and rid the body of excess water. Examples: Burdock, Dandelion, Juniper

Emetic
These herbs induce vomiting. Examples: Impecacuanha, Lobelia, Squill

Emollient
Emollients are applied externally to soothe and protect the skin. Examples: Comfrey, Fenugreek, Marshmallow

Expectorant
Expectorants help eliminate excess mucus in the respiratory system. A stimulating expectorant will irritate bronchial tissue, thereby provoking a cough to break up the phlegm. A relaxing expectorant will dilate and soothe the bronchial tubes, causing mucus to thin for easier expulsion. Examples: Aniseed, Coltsfoot, Thyme

Hepatic
Hepatic herbs fortify the liver and increase bile flow. Examples: Dandelion, Goldenseal, Wild Yam

Hypnotic
These herbs do not induce a hypnotic state, but rather are powerful sedatives which induce a restorative sleep. Examples: Californian Poppy, Hops, Valerian

Hypotensive
These herbs regulate high blood pressure. Examples: Garlic, Hawthorn Berries, Yarrow

Laxative (Aperient)
Laxatives stimulate bowel movement. Examples: Blue Flag, Cascara Segrada, Rhubarb Root

Nervine
These herbs regulate the nervous system either through a stimulating or relaxing effect. Examples: Kola, Skullcap, Saint-John's-Wort

Pectoral
Pectorals aid and strengthen the respiratory system. Expectorants may be considered pectorals. Examples: Comfrey, Elecampane, Licorice

Sedative
Sedative herbs reduce stress and soothe the nervous system. Anti-spasmodics, hypnotics,and nervines are often considered for similar disorders. Examples: Cramp Bark, Lady's Slipper, Passionflower

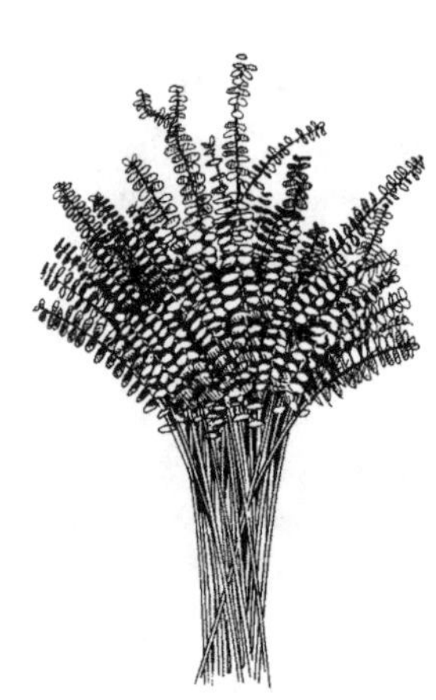

Stimulant

Stimulants increase energy, circulation and invigorate physiological functioning. Examples: Cayenne, Ginseng, Wormwood

Tonic

Tonics stimulate overall health by increasing circulation and improving the absorption of vital nutrients to individual organs. Most tonics are specific to a particular body system such as the nervous system, heart, stomach, liver, biliary, or reproductive systems. Examples: Agrimony (stomach), Hawthorn (heart), Sassafras (liver)

Vasodilator

These herbs dilate blood vessels for increased circulation. Examples: Feverfew, Gingko, Siberian Ginseng.

Vulnerary

When applied externally, these herbs aid in the healing of wounds. Vulnerary herbs often have astringent or demulcent properties. Examples: Burdock, Goldenseal, Sage

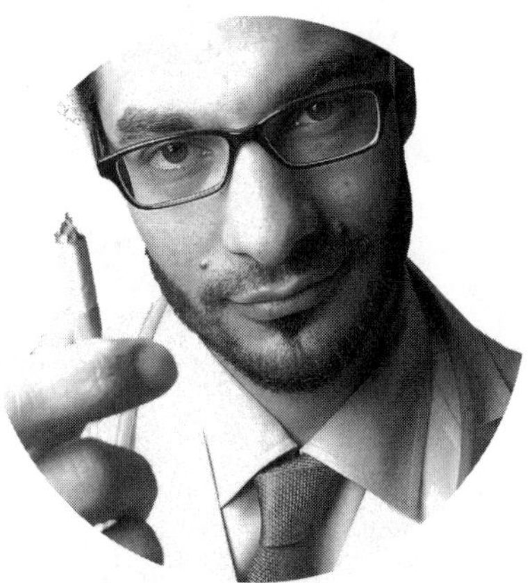

"Nicotine is an awful curse. It strains the heart and drains the purse."
KT Sarma

5 TO SMOKE OR NOT TO SMOKE?

Tobacco Companies Race to Control Vaporization Technology

Smoking is one of the most primitive ways to experience an herbal substance. Native Americans have chewed and smoked tobacco and other plant material for thousands of years. In 1492, Europe was introduced to the herb after Columbus sailed to America and, although its use wasn't popularized until the sixteenth century, it then became an integral cash crop to the colonies of the "new world". In fact, tobacco was so instrumental to the economy of the time that it was a base of currency and was, briefly, as valued as gold. Slowly, tobacco use grew from snuff and pipe smoking to cured leaves and machine-rolled cigarettes in the post-Civil War era. For a time, tobacco users were oblivious to the negative effects of smoking. European doctors even prescribed a cigarette or two to alleviate chronic anxiety and improve concentration.

By the early 20th century, however, speculation began to surface in the medical community about the ill effects of smoking. This drew little attention until 1930, when German scientists uncovered a statistically relevant correlation between cigarette smoke and cancer. By 1944, the American Cancer Society began to warn about the possible hazards of smoking, although admitting to lack of causal data.

Yet the general public remained largely uniformed until 1952 when *Reader's Digest* published "Cancer by the Carton". This milestone article speculated the numerous dangers of smoking, vastly impacted public opinion and immediately spurred the scientific community to further research.

It was the first time in thousands of years that human beings were equipped with the knowledge, to reevaluate smoking as an herbal delivery method, and the first time ever tobacco companies felt the financial hit of a concerned public. Certainly, it wasn't the last.

In 1954, tobacco companies united to form the Tobacco Industry Research Council (TIRC), which countered negative health claims in full-page news articles and other PR coups. The tobacco industry began to produce filtered cigarettes and to offer "low-tar" alternatives. The late 1950s came to be known as the "Tar Derby" as companies raced to develop and successfully market lower-tar cigarettes. Eventually it was found that the designs were largely ineffective as they filtered nicotine as well as tar, causing smokers to compensate by smoking more and inhaling more deeply to obtain the same effect.

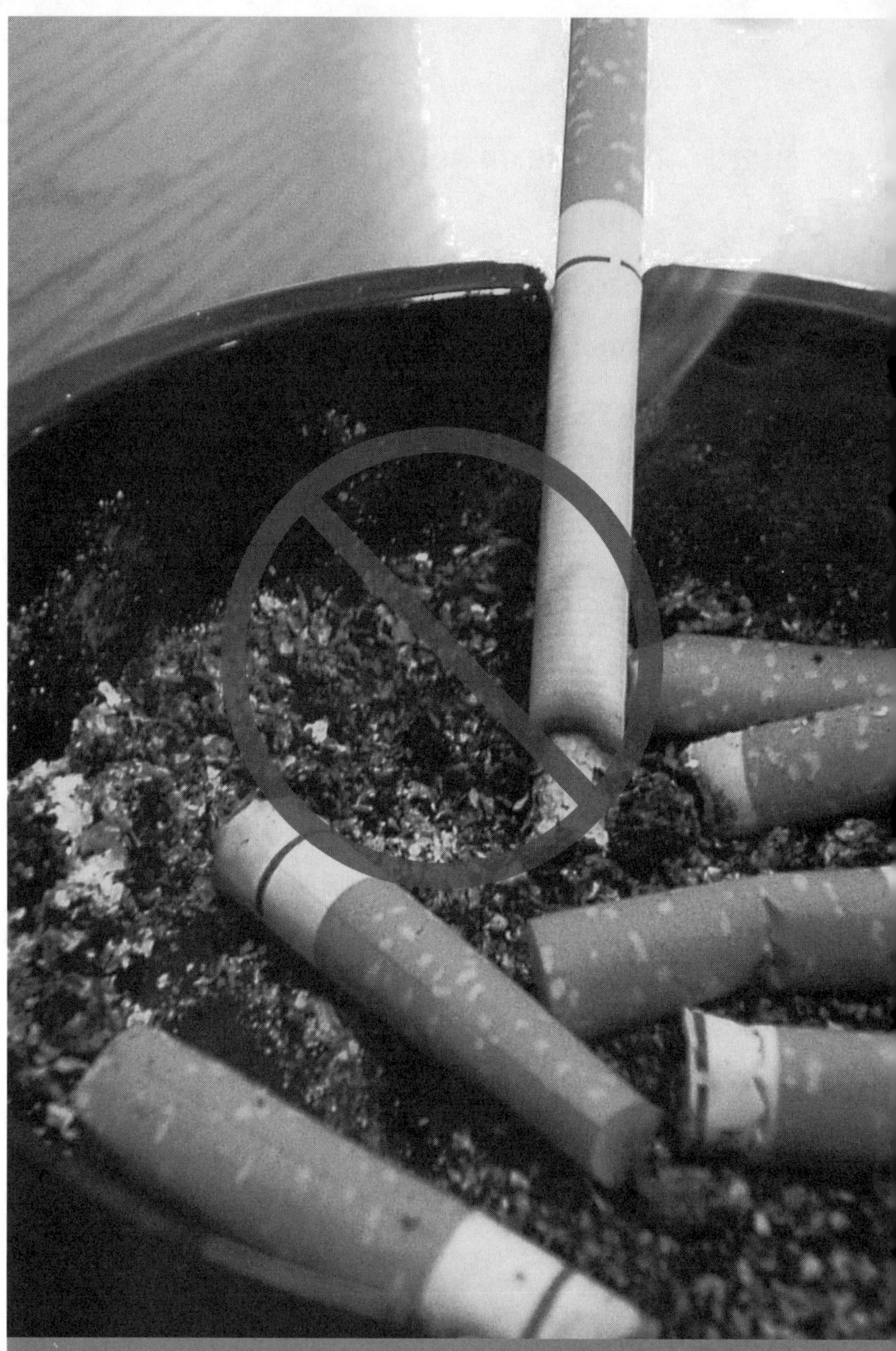

Producing a less harmful cigarette has been a long-running goal of the tobacco industry.

Further efforts to reduce tar focused on three areas:

Synthetics

Tobacco companies explored the potential for synthetic tobacco and tobacco substitutes such as wood pulp. However, composites fell under the FDA classification of "drugs" and were, therefore, mired by regulatory requirements not subjected to the naturally occurring tobacco leaf. In 1977 a few British tobacco companies, able to circumvent USFDA regulations, attempted various synthetic tobacco products, but each suffered from the scrutiny of health groups and were withdrawn after only a few months.

High Nicotine Levels in Filtered Cigarettes

A higher concentration of nicotine would prevent compensatory smoking for the loss of nicotine removed with filters meant for tars.

Selective Filtration

This method involves the development of a more sophisticated filter to discriminate and extract the four known carcinogenic compounds: nitrosamines, aldehydes, polycyclic aromatic hydrocarbons (PAHs), and trace heavy metals. In 1975 Brown & Williamson designed the Fact brand cigarette on the selective filtration method, but the technology was largely ineffective and studies revealed that although the cigarette successfully lowered certain hazardous compounds, it remained dangerously high in others. Fact was pulled from the market after two years.

Each of these techniques proved more difficult than expected. For example, scientists found that removing one harmful agent could inadvertently boost the potency of others.

The technical difficulties, however, were only one of the challenges tobacco companies faced in the quest for a safer cigarette.

CATCH-22

In the early 1970s, the Liggett Group, Inc. began its own search for a safer cigarette in a venture known as Project XA. The project added specialized catalysts to tobacco mixtures in order to neutralize carcinogenic compounds, most especially PHAs. According to the *Wall Street Journal's* Tara Parker-Pope in her book, *Cigarettes: Anatomy of an Industry From Seed to Smoke*, a former tobacco industry lawyer admits that Liggett was pressured to abandon the project by other cigarette makers because "marketing and sale of a safe cigarette could result in infinite liability in civil litigation as it would constitute a direct or implied admission that all other cigarettes were unsafe." In fact, the very tests used to verify the efficacy of the new safer cigarette, tests that utilize a mouse skin-painting technique, were the very tests tobacco company lawyers were in court refuting the reliability of in an effort to stem lawsuits. Eventually, Liggett abandoned Project XA.

This has posed a persistent problem. How can tobacco companies develop and market a "safer" cigarette, without admitting current smoking methods are verifiably "unsafe"? This Catch-22 delayed these companies' research and development of alternative smoking methods until recently when the ill-effects were so specifically and scientifically provable that tobacco giant Philip Morris, after decades of denying any evidence of causality between smoking and cancer, finally admitted that "there is no 'safe' cigarette" and "cigarette smoking is addictive, as that term is most commonly used today.... There is an overwhelming medical and scientific consensus that cigarette smoking causes lung cancer, heart disease, emphysema and other serious diseases in smokers.... Smokers are far more likely to develop serious diseases, like lung cancer, than non-smokers." A section of the Philip Morris website even has suggestions for quitting altogether. RJ Reynolds also addresses the risks of smoking and dedicates a section of its corporate site to "Youth Non-Smoking Programs".

Although lawsuits have erupted furiously, the admission has freed these companies to openly research and develop new smoking techniques. It is an understandably alluring goal. By offering an alternative to smoking, tobacco companies stand to reduce their liability for the wealth of health issues attributed to smoking. In addition, smoking cessation is a huge and profitable industry. For most any company, profit is the bottom line and, although it may seem contradictory, smoking cessation is a logical product expansion for the smoking industry itself. A final incentive to develop healthier means of enjoying tobacco is also tied to profit, though it is an unpleasant actuality. Simply put, a significant percentage of big tobacco's loyal customers die young. This industry challenge no doubt instigated the onslaught of marketing efforts to attract teenage smokers, a strategy that has recently met with much social and legislative opposition. Healthier tobacco products mean longer life-spans, and a larger customer base for a longer period of time.

1988

In this year, RJ Reynolds introduced Premiere, a cigarette made of aluminum capsules containing tobacco. The tobacco, shaped in small pellets, was designed to be "vaporized", in a way, as it was meant to be heated instead of burned. The product produced almost no smoke and was fashioned like a traditional cigarette, although an instruction booklet was required to illustrate how to light it.

Premiere struggled from the beginning however. RJ Reynolds had steeped $800 million in development and battled government health officials who argued the cigarette should fall under FDA regulations as a drug. Another obstacle was consumer preference. Smokers simply weren't used to the taste, and some complained of a residual "charcoal" flavor. RJ Reynolds had anticipated this and estimated that smokers would need two or three packs to acquire the new taste. Most consumers, however, refused to put in the effort, and often quit the brand after a few cigarettes. Less than a year after its debut, Premiere was removed from the market.

1989

Philip Morris followed with Next brand cigarette. This project focused on the addictive qualities of nicotine, and designed ways to remove nicotine, rather than tar, from its new cigarette. Next was marketed as a flavorful and "de-nic" variety and was boasted to be virtually indistinguishable from traditional brands. Critics however, condemned the product for its excessive levels of tar and pointed out that most users would simply smoke more to compensate for the lower nicotine levels.

1996

In the 1990s, science spotlighted the hazards and biological activity of side-stream smoke. RJ Reynolds responded with Eclipse, a smokeless cigarette claimed to reduce second-hand emissions, or environmental tobacco smoke (ETS), by up to 90 percent. Eclipse also claimed to be lower in tar and nicotine. The cigarette works with a heat source of high-purity carbon, surrounded by an insulation layer. Inside the shaft are two rolls of tobacco, one of which is high in glycerin. When heated, the vaporized glycerin particles carry the flavor and active substances of the tobacco into the lung. Reynolds claims that only the heat source and roughly 3 percent of the tobacco actually combusts; however, phytotechnicians who have inspected the spent tobacco of the Eclipse have found it to be dark in color and highly denatured in appearance.

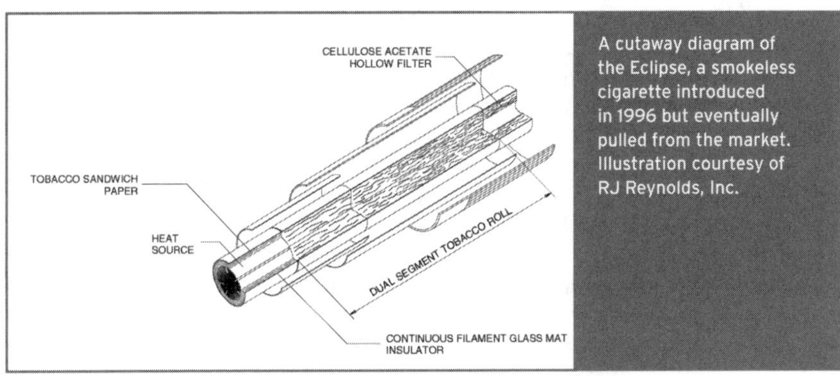

A cutaway diagram of the Eclipse, a smokeless cigarette introduced in 1996 but eventually pulled from the market. Illustration courtesy of RJ Reynolds, Inc.

RJ Reynolds released a careful statement. "We're not making any safety claims whatsoever about Eclipse. Eclipse represents an attempt on our part to provide smokers what they've been asking for," Kevin Verner of RJ Reynolds told CNN, referring to the reduction of side-stream smoke.

Independent studies commissioned by the Massachusetts Tobacco Control Project revealed some disparaging data on the Eclipse. Researchers concluded that nicotine and carbon monoxide are delivered by Eclipse much to the same degree as conventional cigarettes, though several other dangerous compounds are dramatically reduced. The most surprising find was reported by the Roswell Park Cancer Institute. Their research discovered glass fibers in the insulating material of the cigarette's tip. A report published in November of 1998 found 95 percent of Eclipse filters were contaminated with asbestos-like glass fibers. According to Michael Cummings, a senior research scientist at Roswell Park, the glass contamination is a dangerous problem, but one that is easily corrected. The product has yet to be released nationally, where it would likely fall to FDA drug regulations if above findings proved true.

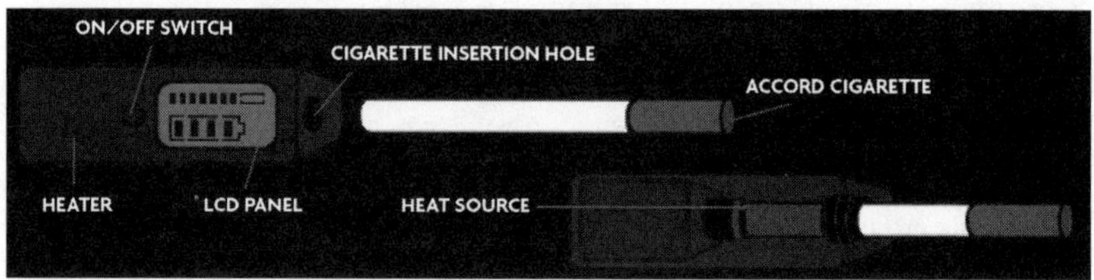

A diagram of the Accord, a device designed by Philip Morris for healthier smoking. Illustration from NOVA Online.

1998

Accord is the most intricate tobacco delivery method to date. The device has been described as "kazoo-shaped", and it is an elaborate cigarette-shaped vaporization system. The device itself is a microchip-controlled lighter that is activated by the user's inhalation. A $40 starter kit includes the lighter device, a battery charger, and a carton of Accord cigarettes. Smokers insert a cigarette into the end of the lighter and, as they puff, the microchip heats one of the lighter's eight coils for a two-second burn. Each coil will facilitate a single puff. An LED display counts down the number of puffs remaining in the cigarette, in the way a camera will mark pictures remaining on a roll of film. The combustion temperature is somewhat controlled and consistently heats to about 950°F. This is much cooler than a traditional cigarette, which yields a temperature of roughly 1,650°F when inhaled. However, this is still above the combustion point and releases catalyzed materials that are not produced with true vaporization. Although, as combustion only takes place as the user inhales, there is no side-stream smoke, and the overall environmental tobacco smoke is dramatically reduced.

Philip Morris makes no formal health claims about the Accord; however, the Society of Toxicology reports that Accord generates 83 percent fewer toxins than a regular cigarette. Test marketing of the Accord has shown consumer resistance to the new smoking

Brown & Williamson's safer Advance cigarette uses its special Trionic filter to reduce tar and harmful toxins. Diagram courtesy of Brown & Williamson Tobacco.

ION EXCHANGE RESIN
TOBACCO SECTION
ACTIVATED CARBON
CELLULOSE ACETATE

Smoking Fact:

A regular smoker between the ages of 35–69 has a 50-percent chance of dying from smoking. (*source: World Health Organization*)

ritual and paraphernalia required. This product has yet to be nationally released.

2000

Not to be left behind, Brown & Williamson recently released Advance — its version of a safer cigarette. Advance implements what is called a trionic filter. A trionic filter uses three separate filtration devices, one each to screen the constituents of smoke in both its physical states, particulate matter (tar), and gas. The third filter strains "semi-volatiles", which are a mix of particles and gas.

According to researchers at Brown & Williamson, the trionic filter substantially reduces tars and noxious chemicals when compared to Lite brands. Advance has met severe opposition, however, based on its healthful claims, which have yet to be supported by independent research.

DIGITAL VAPORIZATION TECHNOLOGY

Although not for lack of effort, tobacco companies have as yet been unable to produce and market a successful non-carcinogenic delivery device for tobacco. The alternatives developed to date have involved at least partial burning of the material, and this may be their most significant weakness.

One innovative company, Star Scientific, Inc., takes a surprising approach to tobacco sales and production by making public health not just a concern, but a priority. Star Scientific publicly endorses all Surgeon General reports on the dangers of smoking tobacco and focuses on the aggressive pursuit of safer tobacco. The company asserts their "corporate responsibility to continue to expand research and development efforts that result in the manufacture of tobacco products that contain as few toxins as is technologically feasible". This is done through a patented curing process which removes what they call Tobacco Specific Nitrates (TSN). Impending products include a series of low-TSN cigarettes in four varieties: Main Street®, GSmoke®, Vegas®, and Sport®. These cigarettes will have 97 percent standard tobacco and only 3 percent of the low-TSN tobacco, due to its limited supply. Star Scientific aims to increase the amount of low-TSN tobacco over time. The company also develops charcoal filters and specially-cured smoke-less tobacco.

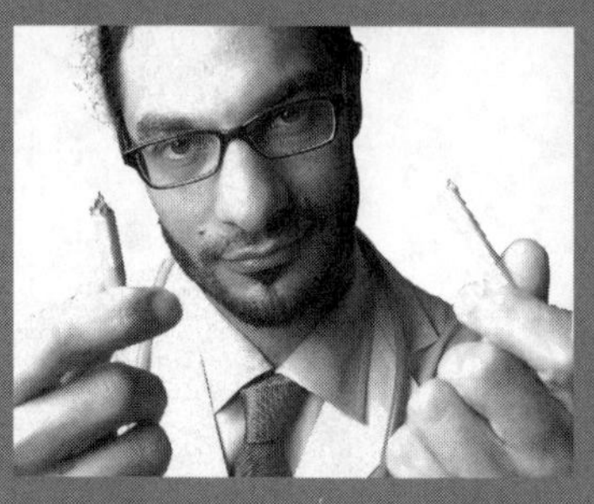

Smoking Fact:

Long-term smokers have a one-in-four chance of developing some type of cancer. (*source: American Cancer Society*)

The difficulties of this endeavor are enormous. Even at the research and development stage, Star Scientific faces a grueling legal climate, and not just from public skepticism and FDA restriction. The industry of Big Tobacco faces a radical and permanent change and competition within the industry is heated, to say the least.

In May of 2002, Star filed suit against RJ Reynolds for patent infringement. In July, Philip Morris filed the same suit against Star for a similar patent. The Morris suit was subsequently dropped for lack of grounds, but the Reynolds suit still lingers in the courts. Even in these fierce times, some cooperation has emerged. Brown & Williamson, for example have entered into a licensing agreement with Star for the curing patent and several smaller companies are in negotiations to the same end.

These mega corporations compete not only with each other but with major pharmaceutical companies for control of the integral patents. Beneath the clamor of these giants, a few smaller players have leapt into the equation. Smaller entrepreneurial companies have developed their own remarkably successful technologies and individual vaporization has sprung to the forefront of applicable alternatives to smoking tobacco.

Vaporizing tobacco completely prevents the formation of toxins which are necessarily created by the combustion of smoking. These toxins are utterly absent in vaporization. A personal vaporizer allows the consumer to control the dosing in a way impossible with smoking. With the cultivation of this technology, inhalation devices may become more "cigarette-like" in design, but over time consumers will likely grow accustomed to the slightly different ritual involved with using a vaporization device. Eventually, rather than designing vaporization devices that mimic the ritual of smoking, technicians will be free to design devices based on maximum efficiency, portability, and convenience.

The absence of smoke makes vaporization an ideal on-the-go option for buses, airplanes, and public buildings. Nothing currently comes close in terms of portability and ease of use while creating little disruption and zero health risk to others.

CESSATION

The physical dangers of smoking obviously cannot be ignored. Increased risks include cardiopulmonary disease, respiratory ailments, and various cancers. All of these risks stem from the compounds created when the tobacco leaf is ignited and not from the properties of tobacco alone.

Advanced filtration devices and partial burning of the tobacco may reduce certain health risks, but the main hazardous compounds remain. Vaporization offers an alternative to the harsh effects of combustion, and also may be a helpful stepping stone toward cessation of nicotine use altogether.

But to many smokers, quitting is a long and difficult proposition and the dangers, although well recognized, often lack certainty, immediacy, and the personal relevance needed to prompt the dedication to quit. So let's take a look at some bare-bones basics about the realties of smoking.

Why Quit?

First off — death. Listen to this: smoking kills more people than illicit drugs, AIDS, alcohol, car accidents, murders, suicides, and fires combined![1] It is the number-one cause of preventable death in developed countries. The American Lung Association reports that smoking causes one in five deaths in the United States. That would be more than 440,000 deaths per year. What does this mean for you? Well, if you're a regular smoker between the ages of 35 – 69, you have a 50-percent chance of dying from smoking![2] Before you die, however, you're likely to develop any of several chronic, debilitating and or deadly diseases.

Emphysema: "When you can't breathe, nothing else matters."

This slogan from the American Lung Association exemplifies the severity of lung disease. Emphysema is only one of the respiratory diseases associated with smoking. But how many smokers understand what emphysema is and what it can do?

Emphysema destroys lung tissue, specifically the alveoli, or air sacs, leaving gaps or holes in your lungs. Your lungs will lose their elasticity and you'll no longer be able to move air in and out. If you develop this disease, your symptoms will include:

- Chronic coughing and wheezing
- Shortness of breath
- Fatigue
- Anxiety
- Bluish skin-tone due to a lack of oxygen in the blood
- Heart problems
- Depression

There is no cure for emphysema. Your course of treatment may include portable oxygen, oral medication, or lung reduction surgery where they will actually remove a percentage of your lung mass.

Cancer

Cancer is when malignant cells divide uncontrollably, thereby spreading and destroying healthy tissue. Lung cancer is the most obvious smoking-related cancer, but smoking can also provoke cancers of the throat, nose, mouth, larynx, esophagus, kidneys, pancreas, stomach, and bladder. Long-term smokers have as much as a 30-percent chance of developing cancer.[3] The symptoms of lung cancer include:

- Chronic coughing
- Constant chest pain
- Coughing up blood
- Swelling of the neck and face
- Wheezing, shortness of breath
- Repeated problems with pneumonia or bronchitis
- Loss of appetite
- Fatigue

Cancer treatment includes: surgery where part of all of a lung may be removed, chemotherapy, radiation therapy, or laser therapy for especially small tumors. Side effects of these treatments include swelling, chronic pain, fatigue, nausea, and hair loss. Many patients need several weeks or months to recover.[4]

Cardiopulmonary Disease

Coronary heart disease is the most prevalent form of heart ailment associated with smoking and refers to a diminished blood flow and oxygenation to the heart. Other dangers include the raised potential for aneurysm and stroke. Cardiopulmonary problems can be the quickest killers of all smoking-related diseases.

Now that we've examined some of the grim realities of smoking-related diseases, let's look at the fundamentals needed to quit.

The Good News

People can and do quit. Nearly three million smokers kick the habit every year in the United States. If you're one of the millions who've attempted to quit and failed, don't worry — you're not alone. Many of these successful "quitters" succeeded only after several attempts. Don't give up!

Dr. Kleinman outlines the immediate health benefits of smoking cessation in his valuable book, *The Complete Idiot's Guide to Quitting Smoking*. Within 24 hours, your chances of heart attack decrease! After 48 hours, your nerve cells have begun to restore and smells and tastes sharpen. After 72 hours, breathing eases and, after several weeks, energy rises, and physical activity is easier and coughing and congestion abates. A single year of abstinence form smoking cuts your risk of heart disease in half. After five years, your chances of lung disease are halved as well.

Other benefits of smoking cessation include a healthier atmosphere — you're no longer foisting second-hand smoke onto those around you, including children, family, and friends. Also, those who quit smoking report a boost in their finances as they not only save on cigarette purchases, but take fewer sick days and are generally more productive at work and at home.

Tips for Quitting

- Make a list of your reasons for wanting to quit. Be as specific as possible. Hang this list somewhere you'll see it every day.
- Remember, withdrawal effects are temporary.
- Set a target date and keep a calendar. Celebrate each smoke-free week!
- Tell friends, family and co-workers that you're attempting to quit. Not only will they lend support when the going gets rough, but a sense of obligation may keep you from giving in.
- Don't go it alone! A majority of those who successfully quit smoking do so with the help of a smoking cessation aid.

CESSATION AIDS

Prior to the refinement of digital vaporization therapy, the choices for smoking cessation aids were rather limited. These aids are still available and widely used. Some are effective, some are not. Most have significant drawbacks.

Smokeless Tobacco

Some smokers make the mistake of switching from cigarettes to smokeless tobacco under the assumption that it is healthier than smoking. It's not. Smokeless tobacco is addictive and, because of chemical additives, highly carcinogenic. Additives include formaldehyde, hydrocarbons, and lead. Those who chew are at higher risk for gum disease, lowered bone density and cancer of the mouth, tongue, cheek, lip, and throat. The most critical problem is the risk of leukoplakia, a cancer which begins as a white core in the mouth, often mistaken for a callus and ignored. According to smoking cessation expert Dr. Lowell Kleinman, leukoplakia is found in more than 50 percent of those who use smokeless tobacco.

Rather than a cessation aid, smokeless tobacco replaces one addiction for another with comparable health risks and equally severe withdrawal symptoms.

Nicotine Replacement Therapies

Nicotine replacement therapies (NTRs) fortify the body with decreasing doses of nicotine. The objective is to supply just enough of the substance to prevent withdrawal symptoms while not enough to maintain the addiction. NTRs should not be used by anyone with diabetes, stomach ulcers, heart disease, asthma, high blood pressure, kidney dysfunction, or liver disease. This therapy is often completed in about six months. According to Kleinman, NTRs can as much as double one's chances of quitting for good.

Several methods of NTRs are available today. Each has benefits and drawbacks and the choice of a cessation aid is often a personal one. Use this as a guide and consult your the choice of a cessation aid is often a personal one. Use this as a guide and consult your physician to determine which therapy is right for you.

Transdermal Patch

Transdermal patches adhere to the skin much like a bandage. Nicotine is delivered in a continual dose and is available in decreasing potency. The patch must be changed daily and eventually substituted with lower-dose patches until the withdrawal symptoms have gone. The site of application should be rotated each day to minimize the redness and skin irritation that erupts on the area of contact. This irritation actually signals a waste of the nicotine as it diffuses over the surface of the skin. Some users also suffer nightmares with the patch as a result of the unfamiliar experience of receiving nicotine throughout the night. This can easily be solved by removing the patch at night. Additional side effects may include nausea, headaches, and dizziness, all of which may be attributed to either withdrawal symptoms or to an overdose of nicotine from the patch. Precise dosing is not possible. Trial and error may result in added discomfort, but when applied correctly the patch affords many an effective boost to their cessation efforts.

Nicotine Chewing Gum

Requires a specific chewing motion, slow and controlled, to prevent a burst of nicotine, which can cause a tingling sensation and dizziness. Users are advised to chew 10 or 20 times and then "park" the gum in a certain area of the mouth, and then periodically chew again. The gum's "parking space" should be rotated as burning or gum irritation may occur. If incorrectly chewed, the user may experience a rush of nicotine, causing nausea, dizziness, and belching. Additionally, the user must be very careful not to swallow while chewing as the nicotine is ineffective through the digestive tract and may cause heartburn or nausea. Precise dosing is also a problem with nicotine gums, and the user may have to chew 20 – 30 pieces a day for the desired effect. When carefully used, nicotine gum aids many people to stave off withdrawal and quit smoking for good.

Nasal Spray

This NRT is available only by prescription. The nicotine-infused spray must be used for 16 – 80 doses per day. The inhaler must be careful not to inhale during the spraying as the nicotine needs to be absorbed through the nasal lining. This is an awkward method, though effective if administered properly.

Nicotine Inhaler

The inhaler is available by prescription only and works similarly to the nasal spray, except the nicotine is absorbed through the lungs. The inhaler is convenient, shaped like a cigarette and easily portable. It has replaceable cartridges that provide roughly 20 minutes of inhaling. A typical user will go through 6 – 16 cartridges per day at a cost of about $25 per week. Common side effects are local irritations in the throat and mouth, coughing, and upset stomach.

Vaporization

> **Digital vaporization technology currently offers by far the most promising technique for both smoking cessation and a more healthful tobacco delivery.**

Digital vaporization technology currently offers by far the most promising technique for both smoking cessation and a more healthful tobacco delivery.

Vaporizing pure tobacco, rather than a synthetic nicotine extraction, gives your body the substance in the form to which it is accustomed. The rapid onset allows for specific incremental control over the amount of nicotine entering the system. This prevents many of the side-effects of other NRT's because with vaporization one can montior nicotine levels during the inhalation process and thereby prevent the ill-effects of over-dosing. Air2 offers NicoHale, which offers pure tobacco leaves in a mesh disk ready for vaporization. This gives the user a quick and precise dose of nicotine without any of the carcinogenic byproducts of smoke. It gives the rich flavor of tobacco in a warm bust of air. It is important to note that tobacco is pure and unaltered, unlike the chemical nicotine synthesized for other NTR therapies. NicoHale's nicotine dosage is carefully adjusted by the quantity of tobacco in each disk, which are available in successively lighter doses as part of a carefully designed cessation program. This is a natural and easy-to-implement system that can be followed a personalized pace. The Vapir is needed to use the disks, but Air2 offers a rebate system whereby upon completion of the program the entire cost of the vaporizer is refunded as a mail-in rebate.

Antidepressants

Buproprione

Certain antidepressants such as buproprione (brand name Wellbutrin or Zyban) have been prescribed to aid smoking cessation. These medications prevent withdrawal symptoms by attaching to the actual nicotine receptors in the brain. Side-effects often include dry mouth, agitation, skin rash and sleep disturbance. Unlike NRTs, the user will smoke for the first two weeks while taking buproprione, until the level of medication builds in the blood. Twelve weeks is usually sufficient for successful cessation.

Alternative Methods

These methods have met with success and have plenty of anecdotal evidence to attest to their efficacy. However, little scientific evidence exists supporting these methods as viable cessation aids.

Hypnosis

Many smokers have found success with this approach and it is an atttractive alternative to methods which require medication or nicotine dosing. For those who truly wish to quit and feel that their difficulty stems primarily from lack of will power, hypnosis may be a good choice. The sessions can get costly, however, and no evidence exists as to the efficacy of hypnosis in the long term.

Acupuncture

Acupunture is an ancient Chinese practice that stimulates balance and self-healing by tapping into the body's energy channels, or meridians. Slim needles are strategically placed to undo any blockages that may be creating an imbalance in the body's energies. There usually are no side effects, yet the procedure may be uncomfortable. There also is little evidence that is an effective smoking cessation aid uness it is combined with other methods. See our reference page for smoking cessation resources.

TOBACCO LEGISLATION TIMELINE

Early 1960s	The first substantiated evidence against smoking begins as political pressures and growing scientific evidence incites the formation of the Surgeon General's Advisory Committee on Smoking and Health.
1964	Surgeon General's Advisory Committee releases "Smoking and Health", a 387-page report that finds an irrefutable causal relationship between smoking and lung cancer. This report is the first to cite specific carcinogens contained in smoke such as cadmium, DDT, and arsenic.
1965	Surgeon General's warnings become mandatory on all packs of cigarettes sold in the country.
1971	All broadcast advertisements are banned.
1982	The Surgeon General announces the potential for second-hand smoke to cause lung cancer.
1984	FDA approves nicotine gum as a "new drug" and smoking cessation aid.
1985	Lung cancer surpasses breast cancer as the number one killer in women.
1986	Brown & Williamson win the largest ever libel case against a news organization. CBS pays $3.05 million to B&W for broadcaster William Jacobson's 1981 commentary in which he accused B&W of luring kids to smoke through intentionally sensational advertising.
1990	Smoking is banned on interstate buses and flights under 6 hours.
1994	Mississippi files the first of 22 lawsuits against tobacco companies as retribution for millions of dollars in Medicaid expenses for smokers.

1995 Liggett Group settles with five states for over $10 million in Medicaid expenses for the treatment of smoking-related illnesses.

1995 "Action Against Access." Philip Morris announces this voluntary program designed to prevent youth access to cigarettes.

1996 President Clinton approves FDA restrictions on tobacco sales and advertising to minors. This also gives FDA jurisdiction to regulate cigarettes as a "drug delivery device".

1996 Liggett Group settles lawsuits with another 22 states. They pay $750 million and become the first tobacco company to admit that cigarettes are addictive and can cause cancer.

2000 The Supreme Court rules the FDA has no jurisdiction to regulate tobacco in its current manner. The court asserts that the FDA exceeded its congressionally given authority in attempting to regulate nicotine as a "drug."

"The awareness that health is dependent upon habits that we control makes us the first generation in history that to a large extent determines its own destiny."

Jimmy Carter

6 VAPORIZATION: INTO THE FUTURE

Vaporization technology has experienced tremendous advancement over the past decade. Even seven years ago, the types of vaporization available were crude at-home attempts, even involving kitchen utensils such as large spoons and tin pots. Although based in a solid concept, these attempts lacked the proper technology and implementation to produce the goal of consistent, portable, and pure vaporization. In an incredibly short period of time, however, substantial developments have been this goal a reality and opened the door for so much more.

The current methods of digital vaporization technology, the strict temperature control, exact dosing, portability, and ease of use, allow for exciting new advancements and extraordinary possibilities in several major areas of medicine and health.

Tobacco

One such industry that contributes to and is exceedingly impacted by this technology is, of course, big tobacco. We've examined how tobacco companies have and continue to struggle for a healthier, portable alternative to smoking. Yet, elaborate filters, various types of tobacco, and partial-vaporization products are as close as they've come to date. None of these methods saw commercial success, and in no case were the tobacco companies able to create a viable device that didn't burn at least part of the material. Instead, they marketed devices mainly based upon an inferior hybrid of vaporization and combustion combined.

How could they fail? This is an interesting question. With such pressure and enormous sums of money revolving around the discovery of just such a product, how could not one, not two, but all three major multi-million dollar corporations have been so off-the-mark?

Vaporization scientist Stephen Kessler recognizes one reason to be the legal position of tobacco companies regarding the health issues of smoking. As briefly discussed in the Addendum, tobacco companies such as Philip Morris and RJ Reynolds were in court arguing against any causal correlation of smoking and various heath problems. Any public development and marketing of a "healthier" cigarette would imply admission that regular cigarettes are unhealthy. In these cases, it is surmised that the company would create and patent a workable idea, with the express purpose of not developing the product. In this way, the company would retain control of the technology, thereby preventing the development of successful product which might challenge Big Tobacco's health claims and rival market domination of current cigarettes.

Kessler cites design limitations as another reason for tobacco companies' failure to create a viable vaporization device. Big Tobacco concentrated solely on designs that mimicked the basic smoking ritual. Marketing concerns held that consumers would be uninterested in something new and different, such as a re-fillable tobacco device. Re-fillable tobacco products also put the companies at risk for a loss of market share, as competitors both large and small would be able to provide the simple product of pure, loose tobacco leaf. No matter the motives, a cigarette-like design for vaporization purposes simply yields high cost and low performance.

Another likely reason for Big Tobacco's resistance to develop a truly feasible and rewarding smoking alternative is the volumes of potential lost customers who would use vaporization devices to quit their habits altogether.

Smoking Cessation

Perhaps the single largest and most immediate effect of a perfected vaporization method is smoking cessation. Smoking causes more than 440,000 deaths and over $75 billion in direct medical costs in the United States each year. Most striking is the fact that these diseases, these deaths are entirely *preventable*. So why don't people stop? The answer is: many simply can't.

Nicotine withdrawal symptoms peak 24 to 48 hours after cessation and can last from 3 days to 4 weeks. Intense cigarette cravings can last for months. Smokers who typically smoke at least 15 cigarettes per day or who smoke their first cigarette of the day within 30 minutes of waking are likely to experience nicotine withdrawal symptoms and to find quitting unnerving, distressing, and physically and emotionally difficult.

Relapse rates for smokers are extremely high. Sixty percent of those who have quit return to smoking after three months of cessation, and 75 percent return to smoking after six months. These numbers roughly equal the relapse rates for heroin and alcohol addiction. Nicotine is difficult to beat, and for many it's nearly impossible without help. Until now, there has been little to help smokers safely wean themselves from nicotine, much less enjoy nicotine without the cancer-causing agents involved in smoking.

Vaporization offers the first viable, affordable alternative to smoking. It also fills a significant gap in the smoking-cessation industry and offers an instrumental tool by which to incrementally reduce nicotine intake over a long period of time. Digital vaporization technology is the first significant product to enter the smoking industry in more than fifty years.

Digital vaporizers now offer the ability to release nicotine in a controlled form that can be inhaled. Because they release the natural combinations of active herb elements directly from the plant, the method is more pure and much easier on the body than the absorption of synthetic nicotine. In the form of transdermal patches, chewing gum, or inhalers, synthetic nicotine provokes a harsh and unnatural reaction in the body. Smokers have introduced the same chemical combinations, derived from tobacco itself, into their bodies for as long as decades. The introduction of a chemically isolated and altered chemical is often an abrasive addition to an already taxed system. Vaporization is the best, and most natural way to quit.

> **"Health is my expected heaven."**
> **John Keats**

Over time, as significant numbers utilize vaporization as either an alternate means to enjoy tobacco, or as a gateway to quit smoking altogether, the medical and health care industries should feel the ease of a burden they've carried for decades — namely the disproportionate ill heath and premature death caused by smoking.

VAPORIZATION IN THE MEDICAL COMMUNITY

Miraculous achievement has erupted in the synthesization of medications over the past few years. Biotechnological advancements are astounding and pervasive. However, medications run the risk of being wasted. Vaporization may be the key to the delivery of certain medications. In recent years, biotechnology has developed and synthesized more medications than ever before. However, these new drugs are often "macromolecule" medications, meaning they are derived from proteins or peptides that have a larger molecular structure than most medications. The oversized molecules limit the methods of drug delivery, and a search has been on for a viable alternative to current delivery methods, each of which carries significant disadvantages.

Oral Delivery: These proteins and peptides are easily digested and, when taken orally, often fail to reach the bloodstream at all. Additionally, oral delivery has a slow onset because it takes an indirect route to the bloodstream, as it is not absorbed until it traverses the digestive tract and reaches the gastrointestinal system. One advantage of oral delivery is that it is highly convenient and painless for the patient, although because of dissolution in the digestive tract, oral delivery is it is not generally an option for macromolecule drugs.

Intravenous Delivery: IVs have direct delivery into the bloodstream and, therefore, provide a very rapid onset. Also, they can easily transmit larger molecules. However, IVs are inserted through a needle, and require administration by a healthcare professional. They also take time to dose, and require the patient to lie still for the duration of the dosing. This type of delivery is significantly inconvenient for the patient.

Injections: Intramuscular or subcutaneous injections (into the muscle or under the skin) have a slightly slower onset than IVs, as the medication must be absorbed from the injected tissue into the bloodstream. However, needles in general are quite unpopular with patients. A recent survey found that 85 percent of patients desired an alternate method of dosing. They are also inconvenient and may need to be administered by a health care professional.

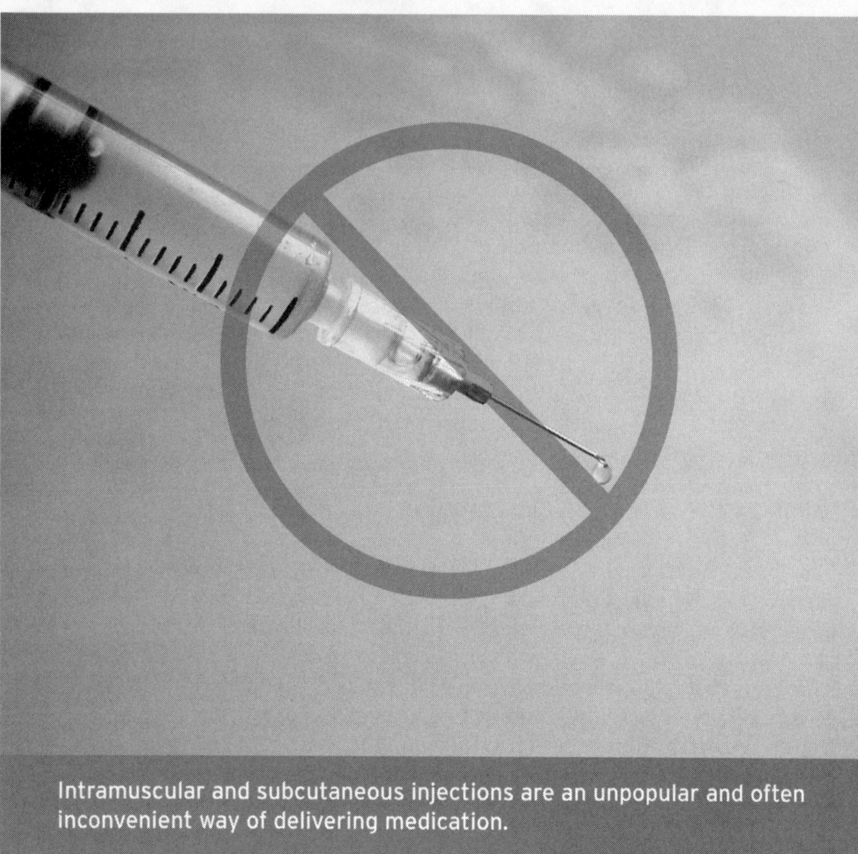

Intramuscular and subcutaneous injections are an unpopular and often inconvenient way of delivering medication.

Transdermal: These gel-like patches apply medication directly to the skin. The onset is relatively rapid, as when absorbed through the skin, the medication reaches the blood immediately. However, irritation often develops, dosing is imprecise as medication can be diffused across the skin and thereby never reach the blood. In addition, the applications are time consuming for the patient.

Nebulizer: A nebulizer is a device that uses pressure to convert specially prepared liquid medication into a fine inhaleable mist. Some nebulizers use an ultrasonic wave that vibrates and breaks the particles into a fine, wet cloud. Nebulizers are often used by asthmatics, as the medication may be applied locally and directly treat respiratory ailments. However, nebulizers can be expensive and are neither convenient nor easily portable.

Advanced Pulmonary Techniques: In the past decade, two major drug delivery companies have emerged. Inhale Therapeutic Systems, Inc. and the Aradigm Corporation each developed technologies for the delivery of existing, FDA-approved medications. These companies especially concentrate on medications with limited delivery options such as insulin and hormone therapies.

Inhale has developed the *Pulmonary Delivery Solution* where powdered forms of medication are dispersed as a fine aerosol. Among other devices, they produce Metered Dose Inhalers, or MDIs. An MDI is a hand-held device with a pump-action spray that delivers medication directly into the respiratory system. However, patients often have difficulty synching their inhalation with the high-powered spray pump. This pump acts with sufficient force to transform the medication to the fine-moleculed mist. Unfortunately, this force is also sufficient to lodge a portion of the medicine in the back of the user's throat, causing irritation and significant waste of material.

Aradigm currently offers *Aerx*, an electronic, liquid medication inhaler which breaks the liquid into an inhaleable mist at the moment of use, a feature which enhances the shelf life of the product. The Aerx has a digital display and built-in memory to keep track of doses, times, and medications taken. Additionally, Aradigm is developing an inhalation-powered, rather than forced-release inhaler in upcoming products, in an attempt to minimize the amount of medication wasted in the throat.

Additionally, a young, San Diego based company, Vapotronics, Inc. has developed an innovative new system called InJet Digital Aerosol Technology. The method involves liquid medication distributed via disposable patient-specific cartridges in a manner similar to the ink-jet technology of a common desk-top printer. This "thermal droplet ejection" dispenses the medication in consistent droplet sizes specific to each particular medicine, and the users inhale the liquid vapor at their own pace. The most interesting aspect of Injet's technology is their application of digital information, similar to the information enhancements available with digital vaporization. Injet's unit, referred to as a "smart device" will have the ability to capture patient information including medical history, medication dosages, physician and health care providers. Security measures digitally monitor usage and prevent over-medication. The liquid medicines must be clinically prepared for the device which, at the moment, limits its immediate application.

The onset for all these devices is about as rapid as vaporization, as the medication is similarly being absorbed by the lower lung. However, they require specialized medication, which is expensive and extremely limited at the moment, a factor that makes the issue of waste during use of the device especially troublesome.

VAPORIZATION

Vaporization is clearly the easiest, most accessible, efficient, and effective way to administer certain substances to date. Many macro-moleculed drugs can be vaporized without the specific and costly preparations required by other inhaleable methods. Almost all herbs can be vaporized from their natural state. Active elements are absorbed readily through the fine network of bronchia in the lower lung and, instead of a blast of medicine, the user receives a gentle flow of air. Furthermore, because of the almost instantaneous onset, as the substance takes effect, users can monitor their reactions and control dosing on a minute level not possible with any other delivery system, except perhaps an IV.

"You see things as they are and ask, 'Why?' I dream things as they never were and ask, 'Why not?'"
George Bernard Shaw

Diabetics especially suffer from the pain and dosage limitations of injections. Injection has long been the only viable way to administer insulin, and many diabetics require anywhere from 1–5 shots per day. Patients commonly admit to skipping a few doses because of the pain and inconvenience of needles. We are finally at the dawn of a new way.

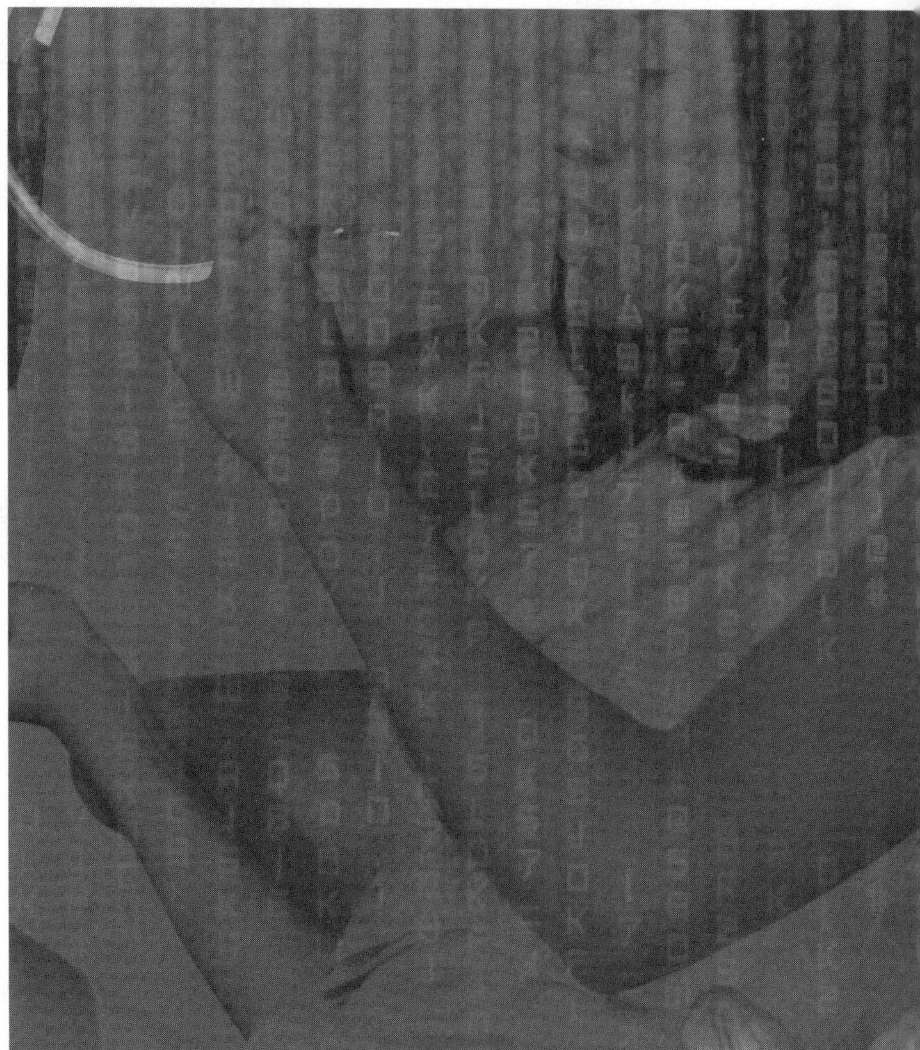

INTO THE FUTURE, AND BEYOND...

Once medical-grade vaporizers hit the market, prescription drugs will never be the same. Inhaleable medication with microchip technology offer endless possibilities. Types of medicines with difficult delivery systems such as injected medicines or oral pain medication will be delivered simply and easily with digital vaporization. Slim little disks will provide instant relief as a simple breath carries medication directly to the blood.

The speed and effectiveness of delivery will change, yes. But poised to change as well is the very process of prescribing medication and purchasing over the counter drugs.

Imagine this...

Let's say you come down with the bronchitis one week before your big vacation to Fiji. You anxiously visit your doctor, who then writes you a prescription for inhaleable antibiotics. You take the prescription to your pharmacy, pick up an electronically coded disk filled with the precise amount of antibiotics. This disk is fully compatible with your own personal vaporizer at home. (At first, you may also need a prescription for a medical-grade vaporizer, but eventually, home-administered medications will be fully compatible with your own, personal vaporizer.)

Your personal vaporizer will have some enhancements over the model currently available in 2002. You will have advanced digital temperature control and powerful microchip technology, which:

- Reads the prescription from the disk and administers the precise amount. The disk is coded to work only with your personal vaporizer and monitors your usage carefully to prevent overdosing.
- Communicates with your doctor to relate your progress in real time.
- Communicates with your health care provider relaying diagnosis, physician, prescription information.

So you take your medication and after three days, you're not yet well. With Fiji on the horizon you call you doctor to voice your concern. He communicates with your vaporizer to strengthen your prescription. Fiji comes, and you feel great. Of course, you need the antibiotics for another three days.

On the plane you easily tote your vaporizer and pull it out to inhale a flavorful mixed-herb disk of chamomile, lavender, and valerian to relax and help you sleep during the flight. You plug headphones into the MP3 jack on your vaporizer to listen to some soothing tunes. Then you lie back and...what's that beeping? It's your vaporizer. You've forgotten to take your antibiotics! Good thing your personal unit was set for auditory reminders. This type of advanced technology makes it quite possible that, even the elderly or the very ill, will never confuse or forget their medication again.

Consider Third World countries who don't have the resources for portable emergency medicines, such as anesthesia. Vaporization offers a cost-effective and highly portable solution. Natural medicines, available and inexpensive, can be used to their maximum effectiveness as their essential oils are released in a pure and direct stream into the blood. Vaporized medicine and herbs may be administered anywhere and in trying conditions such as these, vaporization is more sanitary than other common delivery methods

From here, imagination knows no bounds. Forward-thinking minds, such as those dedicated to the development of this long un-recognized technology, have spoken of endless possibilities including, somewhere in the future, devices equipped to synthesize medications based on downloaded information. Literally, downloadable medication, or downloadable drugs.

And the immediate effects? Foremost, the health care of Americans is set for a radical change. Smoking cessation alone will ease a portion of the health care burden. Holistic approaches to health are more accessible and thoroughly understood than ever before. Naturalistic approaches, especially as enjoyed through vaporization techniques, will enhance the overall health and vitality, and smoking alternatives will boost the health and well-being of millions. Once vaporization is fully available and increasing numbers of people learn about this method, more natural remedies will be studied and prescribed.

The time is now. Digital Vaporization makes it easier than ever to change and avoid invasive and unhealthy life choices. It offers a supreme alternative to the impurities of many processed vitamins and supplements, and of course, to smoking. Mental clarity and physical well being are just two of the benefits of making a lifestyle shift which includes the principles of vaporization outlined in this book and the purity of fresh, unsythesized and untainted herbs. Yet, this is the first step. With your individual participation and advocation of digital vaporization, and its subsequent growth and advancement, we are truly on the verge of a stronger, healthier, more balanced world.

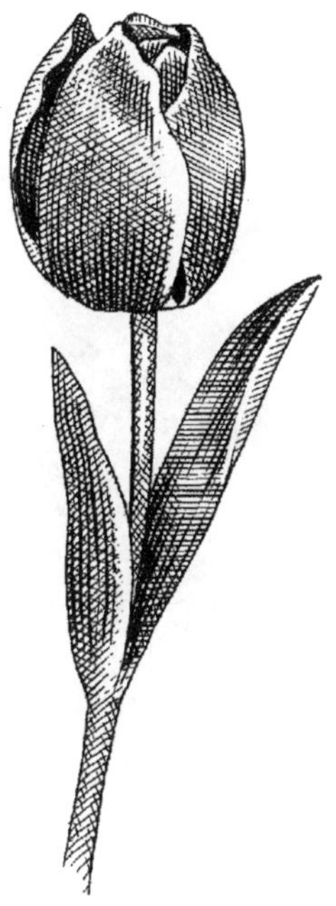

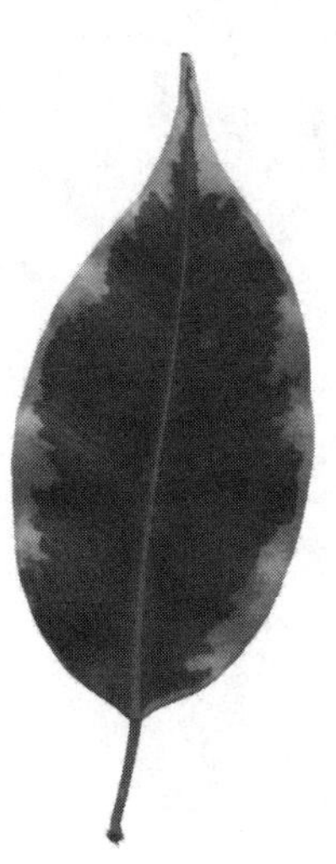

7 PLANT INDEX

Agrimony

Agrimonia Eupatoria

Common names: Church Steeples, Cocklebur, Sticklewort, Philanthropos.

Parts Used: Aerial parts (the whole of the plant above ground).

The agrimony is an erect and downy plant that can grow up to two feet in height and has paired leaves and yellow flowers. The plant is native to Europe and favors wet, marshy climates. Agrimony is a potent astringent helpful with ailments of the liver and the digestive system.

Uses: Topically, agrimony may be used to stem blood flow and heal wounds. Its bitter taste and astringent qualities stimulate digestion and have proved helpful with diarrhea, especially in children. This herb is also widely used to ease appendicitis and, combined with carminative herbs such as corn silk, agrimony is especially effective against cystitis and urinary incontinence.

Actions:
- Astringent
- Digestive Tonic
- Vulnerary
- Cholagogue
- Hepatic

Vaporization Temperature: 200 – 300°F

Warnings: None known.

Aloe Vera

Aloe vera

Common names: —

Parts Used: Gelatinous fluid from leaves.

The aloe vera plant is native to Africa, but has been cultivated, especially as a potted plant, throughout the world. There are several species of aloe, many of which hold therapeutic benefits. However, for the purpose of this book we will deal with the most common aloe: aloe vera.

Uses: The gel from aloe vera leaves provides powerful relief from flesh wounds and burns. When applied topically, aloe will expedite healing and reduce infection. In fact, aloe vera's soothing and astringent properties aid the irritation of many skin conditions including eczema and psoriasis. When taken internally, "bitter aloe", derived from the bitter yellow liquid at the base of the leaves, will cause the colon to contract and acts as a potent laxative.

Actions:
- Vulnerary
- Cathartic
- Astringent
- Laxative
- Anthelmintic
- Hepatic
- External Demulcent

Vaporization Temperature: 350 – 400°F

Warnings: Do not use bitter aloes when pregnant or breast-feeding. Never apply bitter aloes externally.

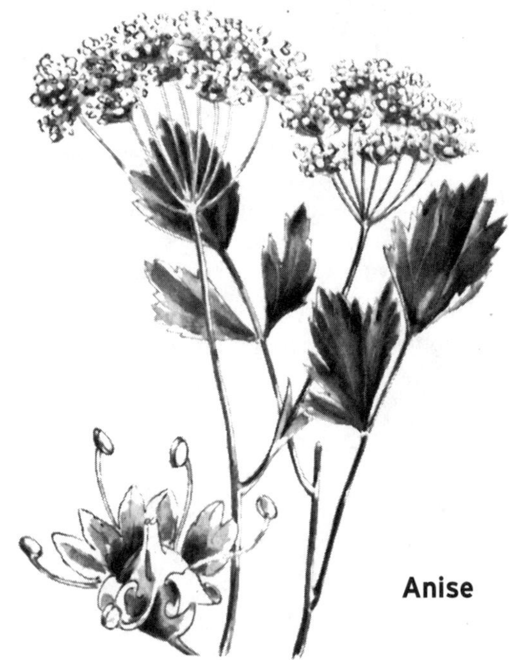

Anise

Angelica

Angelica archangelica

Common names: European Angelica, Garden Angelica, Archangelica Officinalis.

Parts Used: Root, leaves, seeds.

The angelica plant has long hollow stalks, large green leaves, and clusters of small white flowers. It favors a damp atmosphere near running water and can be found in such disparate climates as Europe, the Himalayas, and Siberia.

Uses: Angelica increases circulation, is a strong expectorant for respiratory problems, and an excellent remedy for fever, cold, and flu. Angelica is also useful to diffuse digestive gasses such as colic or general flatulence.

Actions:
- Expectorant
- Anti-Spasmodic
- Diuretic
- Carminative
- Aromatic
- Diaphoretic
- Pectoral
- Respiratory Tonic

Vaporization Temperature: 200 – 300°F

Warnings: Avoid angelica during pregnancy. Excessive use of this herb may cause sensitivity to prolonged sun exposure.

Anise

Pimpinella anisum

Common names: Aniseed.

Parts Used: Seeds.

Anise is a spindly plant, about 18 inches in height with feathery leaves and dainty white flowers. Originating in parts of the Mediterranean, Asia, and North Africa, this plant is now widely cultivated for its seeds, which are valued for both their medicinal and culinary properties.

Uses: Anise seeds are an excellent digestive aid; they quickly reduce gas and bloating and are often used to relieve colic in children. The herb's anti-spasmodic abilities make it useful against menstrual pain and spasmodic-type coughs. **Anise** is also effective against bronchitis and other respiratory ailments.

Actions:

- Carminative
- Pectoral
- Expectorant
- Anti-Spasmodic
- Aromatic
- Galactagogue
- Digestive Tonic

Vaporization Temperature: 300 – 350°F

Warnings: Do not ingest essential oil without professional supervision. Avoid medicinal use of anise during pregnancy.

Barberry

Berberis vulgaris

Common names: Berbery, Pipperidge Bush, Berberis Dumetorum.

Parts Used: Root bark, stem, berries.

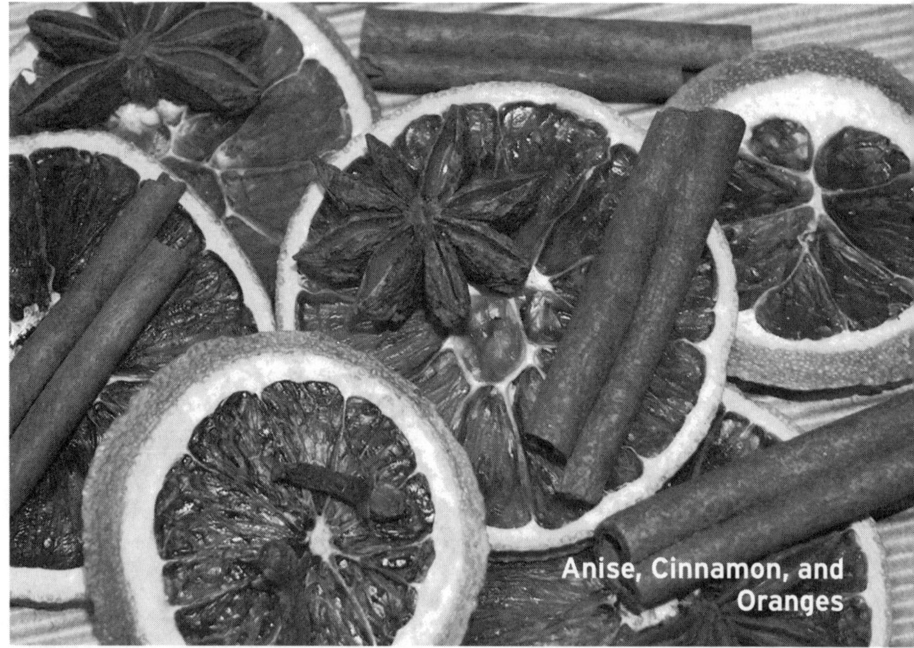

Anise, Cinnamon, and Oranges

Barberry is a thorny shrub with sour red berries. Native to Europe, the barberry has naturalized to North America. In ancient Egypt, barberry was combined with fennel in the treatment for fever.

Uses: Today, barberry is one of the most effective herbs for healing and invigorating liver function and enhancing the flow of bile. The herb's astringent properties soothe and mend intestinal ailments. In fact, barberry is a potent tonic for the digestive system as a whole. Additionally, barberry is a powerful anti-bacterial and has been utilized to fight malaria and has an exceptional ability to reduce enlarged spleen. Studies are currently being conducted on barberry's alkaloids, many of which are thought to inhibit carcinogenic activity.

Actions:
- Astringent
- Digestive Tonic
- Cholagogue
- Hepatic
- Anti-Emetic
- Anti-Bilious

Vaporization Temperature: 350 – 400°F

Warnings: Avoid during pregnancy.

Black Horehound

Ballota nigra

Common names: Stinking Horehound, Black Stinking Horehound.

Parts Used: Aerial parts.

Black horehound grows to three feet in height, has toothed green leaves and pink and white flowers. Black horehound, not to be confused with white horehound, grows throughout Europe, Asia, and North America. The ancient Greeks used this herb to heal ulcers and wounds, and black horehound has long been used to combat convulsions and melancholia.

Uses: Today, black horehound is used primarily to ease nausea and curb vomiting when the cause is in the nervous system, such as with motion sickness, or pregnancy. In addition, this herb is a mild sedative, helps to normalize menstrual cycles, and reduces congestion in the respiratory system.

Actions:
- Anti-Emetic
- Astringent

• Expectorant
• Sedative
• Emmenagogue

Vaporization Temperature: 200 – 300°F

Warnings: None known.

Burdock

Arctium lappa

Common names: Lappa, Fox's Clote, Thorny Burr, Beggar's Buttons, Cockle Buttons, Love Leaves, Philanthropium, Personata, Happy Major, Clot-Bur.

Parts Used: Root, herb, seeds.

Though originally from Europe and Asia, Burdock now grows in temperate climates across the globe. It has broad leaves and round burr-covered fruit. Burdock is considered one of the premiere detoxifying herbs in both Chinese herbal medicine and Western medicine.

Uses: This herb promotes and maintains a state of overall heath throughout the body. The past few centuries have seen Burdock used to treat gout and fevers, and today the herb is widely used to combat any infection or ailment resulting from an overload of toxins in the body. Burdock is helpful for a variety of skin disorders including psoriasis and eczema. External application may treat symptoms of these skin disorders, but internal use of this herb is necessary for healing of the ailment itself. Burdock is typically combined with herbs such as Dandelion to balance its strong cleansing properties.

Actions:
• Antibiotic
• Antiseptic
• Alternative
• Bitter
• Laxative
• Diuretic
• Vulnerary

Vaporization Temperature: 200 – 400°F

Warnings: Fresh leaves may irritate skin.

Caraway

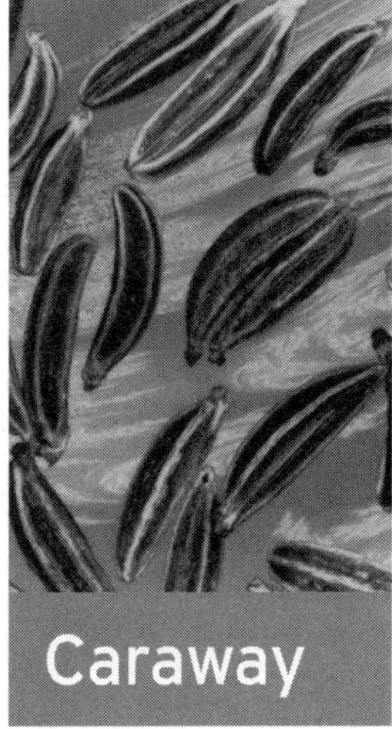

Carum carvi

Common names: Caraway Seed.

Parts Used: Seeds.

Caraway has long smooth stems, feathery leaves, and umbels of small white flowers. Caraway is a wildflower of Europe, North Africa, and Asia, though it is cultivated worldwide. Similar to fennel and anise, caraway seeds are often used in baked goods and ground for culinary oil. Alone or combined with peppermint, caraway is an excellent digestive tonic.

Uses: This herb is highly anti-spasmodic and carminative, thereby relieving intestinal discomfort and digestive ailments, especially flatulence. Caraway is also a strong expectorant and valuable against bronchial congestion and cough.

Actions:
- Carminative
- Anti-Spasmodic
- Anti-Microbial
- Expectorant
- Emmenagogue
- Astringent
- Galactagogue

Vaporization Temperature: 300 – 350°F

Warnings: None known.

Cat's Claw

Uncaria tomentosa

Common names: Una de Gato, Paraguayo, Garabato, Garbato Casha, Samento, Toroñ, Tambor Huasca, Aun Huasca, Una de Gavilan, Hawk's Claw.

Parts Used: Stem bark, leaves.

Cat's claw, named for the claw-like thorns along its stem, is a large woody vine found primarily in the rain forests of the Amazon, and other tropical areas throughout South America. The indigenous tribes of central Peru have long benefited from the use of cat's claw, even in the treatment of life-threatening diseases such as diabetes and cancer.

Western scientists have isolated an important alkaloid in this herb that greatly invigorates the immune system. Clinical studies are underway on the employment of the alkaloid against HIV/AIDS and other immuno-deficiency disorders.

Uses: Cat's claw, like echinacea, with which it is often paired in treatment, has profound effects on the body's ability to fight infection and inflammation. It is an excellent choice against diseases of chronic infections such as chronic fatigue syndrome or HIV/AIDS, and against inflammatory diseases like asthma, and rheumatoid arthritis. In addition, the antioxidant properties of cat's claw are potent enough to suppress the widespread cellular destruction of a chronic degenerative disease such as spina bifida. This herb is useful against the side effects of chemotherapy and may help prevent the formation of cancer cells altogether.

Actions:
- Antioxidant
- Antiseptic
- Anti-Inflammatory
- Cytostatic
- Alternative
- Diuretic
- Hypotensive
- Immunostimulant
- Anthelmintic

Vaporization Temperature: 250 – 400°F

Warnings: Avoid while pregnant or breast-feeding.

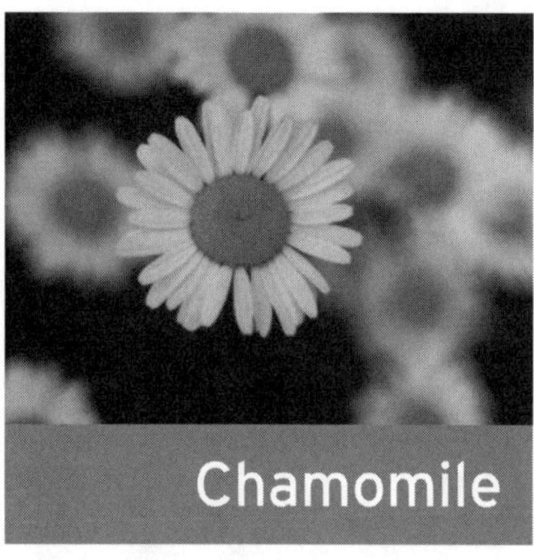

Chamomile

Anthemis nobilis

Common names: Camomile, Roman Chamomile, Garden Chamomile, Ground Apple, Low Chamomile, Whig Plant.

Parts Used: Leaves, flowers.

Chamomile has long stalks, fringed leaves, and yellow and white flowers. This plant was once favored in ancient Egypt, where its powers against illness and fever granted chamomile the honor of dedication to Egyptian gods.

Uses: Chamomile, along with its close relative German chamomile, is widely used in household medicine. It is a gentle and effective relaxant, potent against indigestion and various types of inflammation and, when vaporized, is a potent anti-catarrhal. When applied topically, this herb will promote healing and reduce inflammation of flesh wounds.

Actions:

- Sedative
- Anti-Inflammatory
- Analgesic
- Carminative
- Antiseptic
- Vulnerary
- Anti-Spasmodic
- Aromatic
- Bitter
- Diaphoretic
- Nervine
- Emmenagogue

Vaporization Temperature: 200°F

Warnings: None known.

Clove

Eugenia caryophyllata

Common names: Eugenia Aromatica.

Parts Used: Dried flower buds.

Cloves are the dried, unopened flower buds of the clove tree, which is indigenous to Indonesia, the Philippines and, to a lesser extent, southeastern Africa. Cloves are often used for culinary spice, but the wide array of medicinal properties makes this herb a remarkable medicine as well.

Uses: Cloves have proven beneficial for so many types of ailments that throughout the history of southeast Asia the clove was regarded as a cure-all. This herb is a strong antiseptic and helpful against both infectious diseases and parasites. Its anti-spasmodic abilities ease cough and digestive discomfort, and its stimulating properties enhance both physical and mental agility. Cloves are considered aphrodisiacs in many parts of the world.

Actions:

- Carminative
- Antiseptic
- Stimulant

- Anti-Spasmodic
- Analgesic
- Aromatic
- Anti-Emetic

Vaporization Temperature: 200 – 300°F

Warnings: None known.

Coffee

Coffea arabica

Common names: Caffea, Arabica Coffee, Arabian Coffee.

Parts Used: Seeds.

The name coffee is derived from a province of Abyssinia, Caffa, where the plant is believed to have originated. The coffee plant is an evergreen shrub with thick clusters of white flowers and small red berries. If uncultivated, the coffee plant may grow up to 30 feet in height. It thrives in tropical regions such as the lush climates of Brazil, Mexico and Colombia. Hugely popular today, coffee is often enjoyed when brewed into a hot drink; the use of coffee as a beverage dates back at least as far as Persia in 875. A Persian legend states that a Shepard noticed a liveliness to his goats after they had eaten coffee leaves. He reported this to the prior of the monastery. The monks then tasted the leaves and fruits of the coffee plant and became cheerful and lively at the nightly devotions. Coffee beans may also be ground and vaporized for a pleasurable inhalation and quick benefit of the herbal effects. The primary active ingredient in coffee is caffeine.

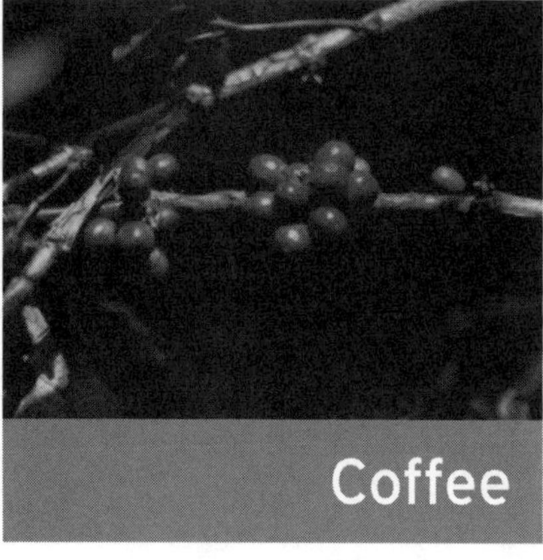
Coffee

Uses: In addition to its rich flavor and fragrance, coffee is an effective stimulant encouraging concentration and energy. Indian medicine has traditionally used coffee to treat migraine, fever, and bowel disorders. Today we know that coffee invigorates blood flow, acts as a diuretic, and is often helpful against diarrhea, inflammations and wounds, especially of the mouth and pharynx. Coffee beans should be finely ground before vaporization.

Actions:

- Stimulant
- Vasodilator
- Diuretic
- Anti-Inflammatory

Vaporization Temperature: 250 – 400°F

Warnings: Those with high blood pressure or heart disease should monitor their caffeine intake.

Comfrey

Symphytum officinale

Common names: Common Comfrey, Knitbone, Knitback, Consound, Blackwort, Bruisewort, Slippery Root, Boneset, Gum Plant, Consolida, Ass Ear.

Parts Used: Root, rhizome, leaf.

Comfrey is a European herb that has naturalized to temperate zones worldwide. The plant has large, deeply-veined leaves and small bell-shaped flowers. Comfrey's common name "Knitbone" demonstrates its astonishing ability to aid in the healing of broken and fractured bones, damaged tendons and ligaments, and to speed the recovery of contused tissue.

Uses: Comfrey is largely used to heal injuries. The herb controls inflammation and encourages bones to "knit" together. Recent research has discovered that Comfrey is rich in the substance allatoin, which encourages cell repair and aids in the healing of tissue and bone. Comfrey is also used to treat digestive ailments and respiratory conditions, and may reduce scar tissue and outbreaks of psoriasis.

Actions:

- Astringent
- Digestive Tonic
- Vulnerary
- Cholagogue
- Hepatic

Vaporization Temperature: 250 – 400°F

Warnings: None known.

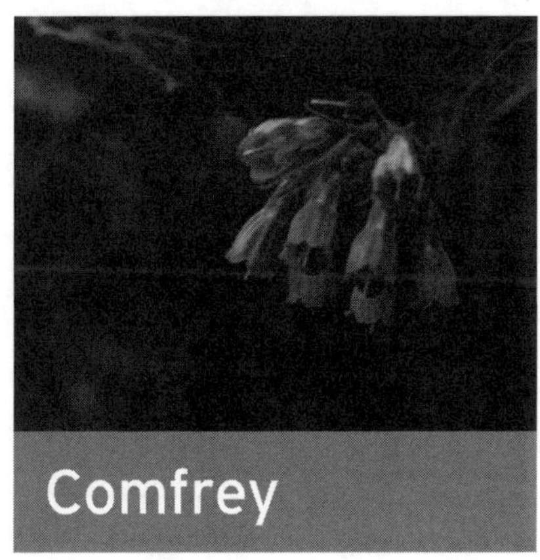
Comfrey

Corn Silk

Zea mays

Common names: Corn Silk

Parts Used: Corn Silk.

Corn silk is the stigmas from the female flowers of maize. These long, thin strands have a sweetish flavor and range in hue from green to gold to reddish-brown. The health benefits of corn have been recognized by Native Americans for thousands of years. Corn silk has a high potassium content and acts as a potent diuretic.

Uses: Corn silk is a valuable remedy for urinary ailments. It soothes the lining of the bladder, reducing inflammation and irritation of the urethra. This herb also suppresses the formation of kidney stones and may help dissolute existing stones.

Actions:
- Diuretic
- Renal Tonic
- Alternative
- Demulcent
- Anti-Lithic
- Mild Stimulant

Vaporization Temperature: 200°F

Warnings: None known.

Couch Grass

Agropyrum repens

Common names: Twitch-grass, Scotch Quelch, Quick-grass, Dog-grass.

Parts Used: Rhizome (underground stem), seeds, root.

Couch grass is a sturdy weed that grows as tall as 32 inches and has long, hollow stems with thin leaves and erect spikes bearing green flowers. This pervasive plant grows in Europe, Northern Asia, Australia and the Americas.

Uses: The diuretic and demulcent properties of couch grass make it an excellent remedy for urinary tract infections. It may also be used to treat enlarged prostate glands and to reduce kidney stones. Juice from the roots has also been used to treat liver ailments such as jaundice.

Actions:
- Diuretic
- Demulcent
- Anti-Microbial
- Anti-Lithic
- Digestive Tonic

Vaporization Temperature: 350 – 400°F

Warnings: None known.

Dandelion

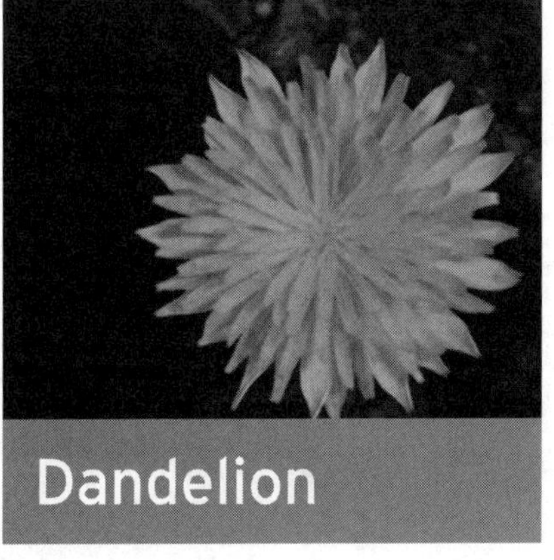

Taraxacum officinale

Common names: Priest's Crown, Swine's Snout.

Parts Used: Root, leaves.

The dandelion weed grows wild across the globe and is cultivated in Germany and France. The leaves of this herb were recorded as a diuretic by Arab physicians in an herbal that dates to the 11th century.

Uses: Dandelion offers an array of therapeutic benefits. The dandelion green has the unique benefit of acting as a strong diuretic without depleting the body of potassium. In fact, dandelion actually increases potassium in the body. The herb also lowers blood pressure, helps remove toxins in the gallbladder, kidneys, and liver, as well as clearing various skin and arthritic conditions such as acne, psoriasis, and gout.

Actions:

- Diuretic
- Anti-Rheumatic
- Cholagogue
- Hepatic
- Laxative
- Anti-Bilious
- Hypotensive

Vaporization Temperature: 250 – 300°F

Warnings: In case of gallstones, consult a physician before the medicinal use of dandelion.

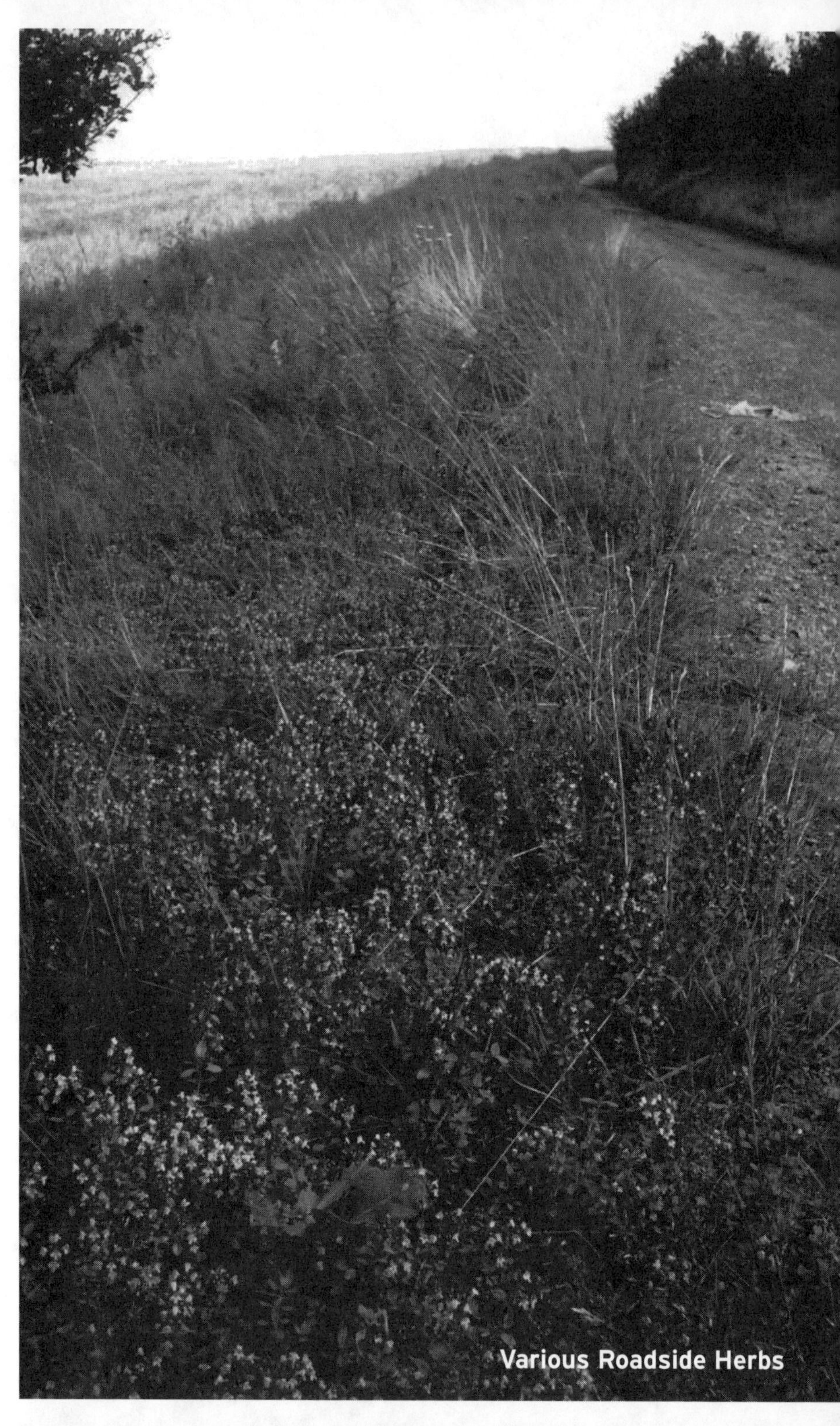

Various Roadside Herbs

Ephedra

Ephedra sinica

Common names: Mahuang, Chinese Ephedra, Epitonin, Cao Mahuang, Mormon Tea, Country Mallow.

Parts Used: Young stems and dried rhizome and roots.

Ephedra is native to West Central China, Southern Russia, and Japan and prefers sandy, rocky climates. This perennial evergreen yields slender green-yellow stalks and each plant contains both stamen and pistils, each residing on separate flowers. The male flowers, housing the pistils, bear plump red cones that resemble berries. Use of ephedra dates back 5,000 years to ancient China. In 2,800 BC, the herb earned placement as one of Sheng Nung's 250 plants in his masterwork: *The Divine Husbandman's Classic of The Materia Medica.*

Uses: Ephedra stimulates the nervous system and acts as an excellent vasodilator. It has long been used against allergies, colds, cough, bronchial congestion, and fever. In fact the two main alkaloids of the herb, ephedrine and pseudoephedrine comprise the main ingredient in cold medications today. Additionally, ephedra acts as a mild stimulant increasing energy and concentration. It is a potent athletic aid as it boosts energy without depleting reserves. Ephedra has also recently become a popular weight-loss aid. There has been some controversy over the safety of ephedra as the herb has been linked to heart failure, and extracted ephedrine in excessive doses have caused several accidental deaths. However subsequent scientific research has proven ephedra safe when taken normally. Ephedra as a whole herb is effective and one must recall the difference between an extract and a whole. As large quantities of extracted caffeine may be problematic, enjoying coffee is quite safe.

Actions:
- Stimulant
- Anti-Inflammatory
- Anti-Spasmodic
- Expectorant

Vaporization Temperature: 250 – 350°F

Warnings: Avoid ephedra while pregnant. If you experience dizziness, severe headache, rapid heartbeat, shortness of breath, or excessive anxiety your dose of ephedra is probably too high. If symptoms persist, seek professional advice.

Evening Primrose

Cenothera biennis

Common names: Tree Primrose, Fever Plant, Field Primrose, Kings Cureall, Night Willow-herb, Scabish, Scurvish.

Parts Used: Bark, leaves.

Evening primrose has red splotches along its stem, creased leaves, and yellow flowers. It is native to North America but has been thoroughly naturalized throughout Europe.
Uses: The main actions of evening primrose are astringent and sedative. The herb has been broadly used to treat whooping cough, and is often helpful with digestive difficulties, high blood pressure, and asthma. When applied externally, this herb benefits skin disorders such as eczema.

Actions:
- Astringent
- Sedative
- Anti-Catarrhal

Vaporization Temperature: 300 – 400°F

Warnings: Epileptics should avoid evening primrose.

Fennel

Foeniculum vulgare

Common names: Fenkel, Sweet Fennel, Wild Fennel

Parts Used: Seeds.

Fennel is a dark feathery plant with small ridged seeds and golden flowers. The plant originates in the Mediterranean and in the Middle Ages was combined with like herbs in an effort to ward off witchcraft and evil persuasion.

Uses: Similar to anise, fennel settles digestion and relieves abdominal bloating. The herb is also an excellent diuretic, and beneficial for bronchial problems, including spasmodic coughs. Additionally, fennel seed is long believed to aid weight loss, enhance vigor, and increase longevity.

Actions:
- Aromatic
- Anti-Spasmodic
- Carminative

• Galactagogue
• Hepatic
• Anti-Emetic
• Diaphoretic
• Expectorant

Vaporization Temperature: 300 – 350°F

Warnings: Limit the medicinal use of fennel if pregnant. Fennel is unsuitable for children under five.

Feverfew

Tanacetum parthenium

Common names: Featherfew, Featherfoil, Flirtwort, Bachelor's Buttons.

Parts Used: Leaves.

Feverfew is common throughout Europe, Australia, and North America. This tall plant has thin stems, broad, branched leaves, and yellow and white flowers resembling the daisy. As its name suggests, this herb reduces fever but is also a valuable remedy for migraine.

Uses: Feverfew's leaves contain parthenolide, a chemical known to prevent migraine headaches. Using Feverfew at the onset of an attack will often prevent a migraine altogether. Small quantities are recommended. Feverfew also aids arthritis and inflammatory discomforts and is helpful to induce menstruation.

Actions:
• Anti-Inflammatory
• Analgesic
• Anti-Pyretic
• Emmenagogue
• Digestive Tonic
• Uterine Stimulant

Vaporization Temperature: 250 – 350°F

Warnings: Avoid feverfew if pregnant. Fresh leaves may cause mouth sores when taken orally.

Fringe Tree

Chionanthus virginica

Common names: Old Man's Beard, Fringe Tree Bark, Chionathus, Snowdrop Tree, Poison Ash.

Parts Used: Root bark, bark.

The fringe tree has dark, elliptical leaves and spindly white flowers. It is native to the United States, especially along the Atlantic coast. This herb was a common Native American remedy for inflammations, mouth sores, and flesh wounds.

Uses: Its diuretic, laxative, and cholagogic properties combine to make fringe tree an excellent liver tonic. It is also useful in treating gall-bladder inflammation and gallstones and, as an appetite stimulant, is helpful in the recovery of chronic illness, especially of the liver.

Actions:
- Liver Tonic
- Cholagogue
- Diuretic
- Laxative
- Alternative
- Anti-Bilious
- Hepatic

Vaporization Temperature: 400°F

Warnings: None known.

Garlic

Allium sativum

Common names: Clove Garlic, Poor Man's Treacle.

Parts Used: Bulb.

Garlic has been described as a "veritable wonder herb". The plant consists of individual bulbs, or cloves enclosed in a white skin. A vastly-used kitchen herb for years, garlic is finally gaining tremendous recognition for its diverse therapeutic properties. Garlic is one of the most diversely beneficial herbs available.

Uses: It is a potent adversary to harmful bacteria, viruses, and parasites. Garlic aids in the digestive process, reduces blood pressure and cholesterol over time, and its volatile elements help combat respiratory infections such as chronic bronchitis, recurrent colds, and influenza. Daily usage is often recommended for this herb.

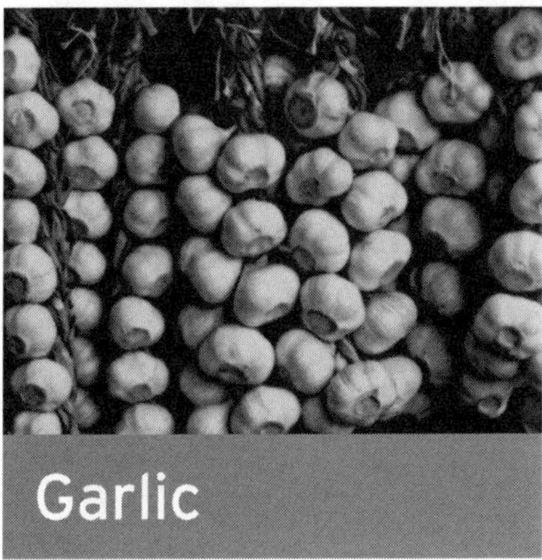
Garlic

Actions:
- Antibiotic
- Antiseptic
- Expectorant
- Diaphoretic
- Hypotensive
- Anti-Spasmodic
- Alternative
- Anti-Microbial
- Anti-Catarrhal
- Carminative
- Cholagogue
- Carminative
- Pectoral
- Rubefacient
- Stimulant
- Vulnerary

Vaporization Temperature: 350 – 400°F

Warnings: None known.

Ginkgo

Ginkgo biloba

Common names: Maidenhair Tree, Duck Foot Tree, Silver Apricot

Parts Used: Leaves, seeds.

Thought to be the oldest tree in the world, evidence suggests the gingko tree first grew over 190 million years ago. The tree is native to China but is also grown in France and South Carolina in the United States. Gingko produces large yellow-green leaves and large, oblong seeds. The properties of this herb have been valued in Eastern medicine for centuries, but only in the past few decades have its advantages been recognized in the west.

Uses: Ginkgo greatly increases blood flow to the brain and overall circulation. Gingko can significantly sharpen mental abilities and combat issues such as declining memory and dementia. It is also known as a preventive, especially in disorders with a compounded and age-related onset such as Alzheimer's disease, or stroke. Furthermore, gingko is an excellent anti-inflammatory agent and has proved useful in treating asthma as well as nerve tissue damaged by swelling related to diseases such as multiple sclerosis.

Actions:
- Antioxidant
- Anti-Inflammatory
- Circulatory Stimulant

Vaporization Temperature: 250–350°F

Warnings: The World Health Organization recommends avoiding gingko for children under 12.

Ginger

Zingiber officinale

Common names: Ginger Rhizome, Ginger Root.

Parts Used: Rhizome

Ginger is native to southern Asia and has naturalized to tropical areas around the globe. The rhizome is a thick, gnarled stem with a brownish-gold hue. In cultivation there are several species of ginger that vary in hue but are similar in effect. Although a popular culinary spice, ginger has been used medicinally for thousands of years.

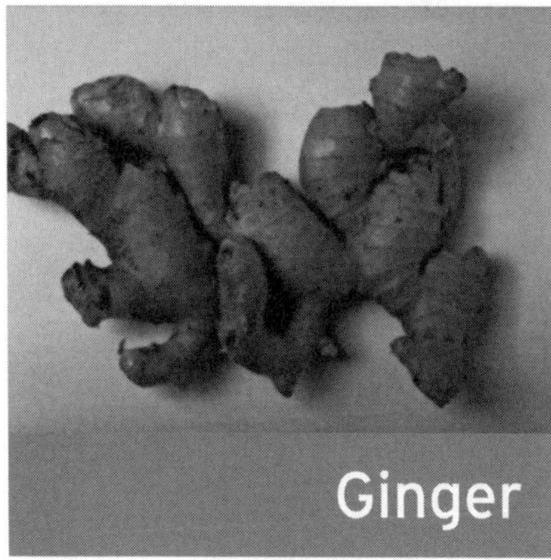

Uses: This highly aromatic herb stimulates circulation, reduces blood pressure, and tones overall health. Ginger alleviates nausea due to motion or pregnancy, and eases gastrointestinal discomfort. It is also helpful against fever, headache, and symptoms of the common cold.

Actions:
- Anti-Emetic
- Circulatory Stimulant
- Carminative
- Aromatic
- Emmenagogue
- Diaphoretic
- Anti-Inflammatory
- Antiseptic
- Rubefacient

Vaporization Temperature: 350 – 400°F

Warnings: Avoid Ginger if suffering from peptic ulcers.

Ginseng (Asian)

Panax ginseng

Common names: Aralia Quinquefolia, Five Fingers, Tartar Root, Red Berry, Asian Ginseng, Chinese Ginseng, Korean Ginseng, True Ginseng

Parts Used: Root.

Ginseng originates in northeastern China, eastern Russia, and North Korea; however, the herb is rarely found in the wild. Though the cultivation process is difficult and the plant requires four years to mature, ginseng is cultivated throughout China, Korea, and the northeast United States. Ginseng is a highly reputed Chinese herb and its benefits are said to date back 7,000 years.

Uses: Recent Asian studies have put science behind millennia of lore in documenting Ginseng's highly "adaptogenic" abilities. The herb contains an astonishingly potent ability to aid the body in adapting to stress. In addition, studies have revealed benefits to the immune system, as ginseng may prevent infections, and improve liver function. Although in Asia it is often prescribed as a stimulant and tonic for the elderly, Western use has found that ginseng, while stimulating the young, has a gentle, restorative effect on the elderly or infirm.

Actions:
- Antidepressant
- Nervine
- Stimulant
- General Tonic

Vaporization Temperature: 350 – 400°F

Warnings: Some experts believe that ginseng is overused in the West, and recommend taking the herb for no longer than six weeks at a time. Ginseng is not recommended for those with heart disease or hypertension.

Goldenrod

Solidago virgaurea

Common names: Verge d'Or, Solidago, Goldruthe, Woundwort, Aaron's Rod.

Parts Used: Aerial parts.

Native to Europe and Asia, goldenrod has naturalized to the Americas. It has spiked branches and golden yellow flowers. This herb is most well-known for its ability to dissolve and remove kidney stones.

Uses: Goldenrod's antioxidant, astringent, and diuretic properties make it an excellent treatment for urinary tract disorders. It has been known to rid the body of stones in the kidney and gallbladder. Additionally, goldenrod is often the first herb prescribed to combat respiratory congestion and bronchial inflammation. Gargling or inhaling vaporized steam is an excellent remedy for laryngitis. This herb is a gentle, effective and safe to use with children.

Actions:

- Antiseptic
- Anti-Inflammatory
- Carminative
- Diuretic
- Antioxidant
- Diaphoretic
- Anti-Catarrhal

Vaporization Temperature: 200 – 300°F

Warnings: None known.

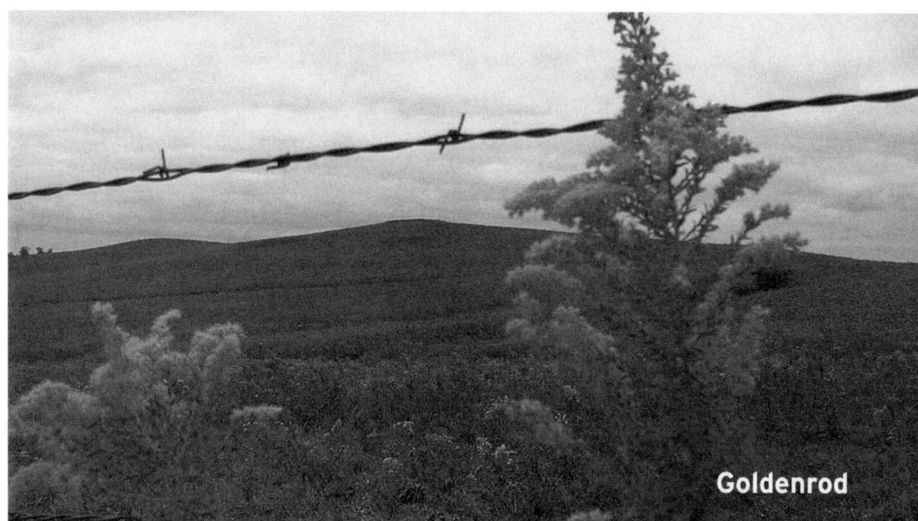

Goldenrod

Goldenseal

Hydrastis canadensis

Common names: Yellow Root, Orange Root, Yellow Puccoon, Ground Raspberry, Wild Curcuma.

Parts Used: Root and rhizome.

Goldenseal is native to the Americas and has been valued by the Cherokee Indians for its ability to heal skin irritations and flesh wounds. The plant itself is unique with broad, thickly-veined leaves, each containing a single bright red inedible berry. The rhizome and roots are brambled and knotty, with a shiny golden hue. Goldenseal is widely used today as an astringent and anti-bacterial remedy.

Uses: Goldenseal is universally accepted as a potent agent against disorders affecting the mucus membranes, especially of the nose, eyes, throat, and stomach. An infusion of goldenseal has proven effective against psoriasis. Additionally, this herb soothes the lining of the stomach, aids digestion, and reduces inflammation of the gut. Goldenseal is also beneficial against gynecological ailments and has been used to stem heavy menstrual flow and stop bleeding after childbirth.

Actions:
- Astringent
- Anti-Catarrhal
- Laxative
- Bitter
- Alternative
- Expectorant
- Hepatic
- Vulnerary

Vaporization Temperature: 350 – 400°F

Warnings: Goldenseal interferes with the ability to absorb certain vital nutrients such as vitamin B. For this reason, goldenseal should be used intermittently rather than for long periods of time.

Gotu Kola

Centella asiatica

Common names: Indian Pennywort, Marsh Penny, Water Pennywort.

Parts Used: Aerial parts.

Gotu kola is a viney plant that grows in the swampy areas of India, Sri Lanka, Madagascar, and South Africa. It is a traditional Ayurvedic herb, often credited with mental and spiritual rejuvenation and used to aid in meditative states. This herb was also a traditional treatment for leprosy and other skin disorders.

Uses: Gotu kola is often regarded as a cerebral tonic for its ability to improve concentration and memory and increase circulation to the brain. It aids in wound healing through its antioxidant properties and encouragement of collagen formation. In western medicine, gotu kola is largely used for its anti-inflammatory action as applied to the treatment of skin disorders.

Actions:
- Cerebral Tonic
- Diuretic
- Anti-Inflammatory
- Sedative

Vaporization Temperature: 200 – 300°F

Warnings: Gotu kola occasionally causes sensitivity to sunlight.

Guarana

Paullina Cupana

Common names: Whitethorn Herb, Hawthorn Tops, Haw, Mayhaw, Mayblossom, Quick Thorn, Hazels, Hagthorn.

Parts Used: Seeds.

Guarana is indigenous to the Amazon basin and thrives in the rain forests of the southern hemisphere. The plant is a sinuous woody vine with large, ribbed leaves and deep yellow fruit.

Uses: Like coffee, guarana contains caffeine and is an excellent stimulant. It enlivens concentration and energy and suppresses appetite. It is used as an energizing tonic, to treat digestive problems, headaches, fever, and circulatory ailments. Guarana is often brewed as a popular weight-loss beverage, but is especially effective when ground and vaporized.

Actions:
- Stimulant
- Tonic
- Diuretic
- Carminative

Vaporization Temperature: 250 – 350°F

Warnings: Those with high blood pressure or heart disease should monitor their caffeine intake.

Hawthorn

Crataegus oxyacantha

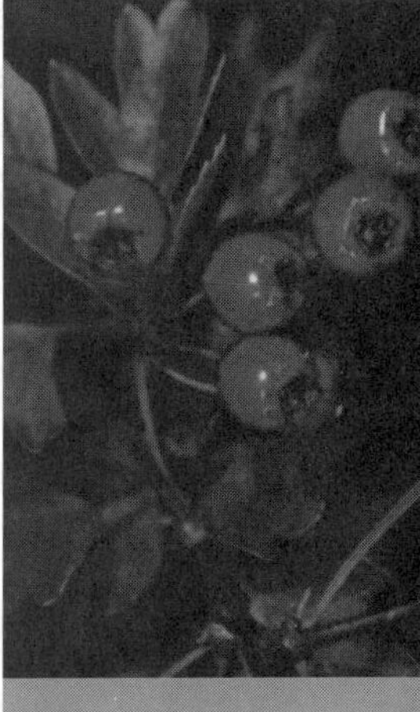

Common names: Whitethorn Herb, Hawthorn Tops, Haw, Mayhaw, Mayblossom, Quick Thorn, Hazels, Hagthorn.

Parts Used: Ripe fruits (berries).

The hawthorn tree grows in most temperate climates of the Northern Hemisphere. It is a full, bushy tree, up to 30 feet tall, bearing ivory-colored flowers and bright red berries. In the Middle Ages, the hawthorn berry was a symbol of hope and used to treat many ailments.

Uses: Hawthorn is an exceptional heart tonic. This herb increases blood flow to the heart and normalizes cardiac function by either stimulating or depressing activity as needed. Hawthorn is used to treat cardiac and circulatory ailments such as angina, palpitations, and mild congestive heart failure. Recent studies in the British Journal of Medicine have shown hawthorn to be an effective agent against high blood pressure, hardening of the arteries, and kidney disease. Combined with gingko, hawthorn berries increase cerebral circulation and improve memory.

Actions:
- Cardiac Tonic
- Antioxidant
- Hypotensive
- Diuretic
- Carminative
- Astringent

Vaporization Temperature: 250 – 350°F

Warnings: None known.

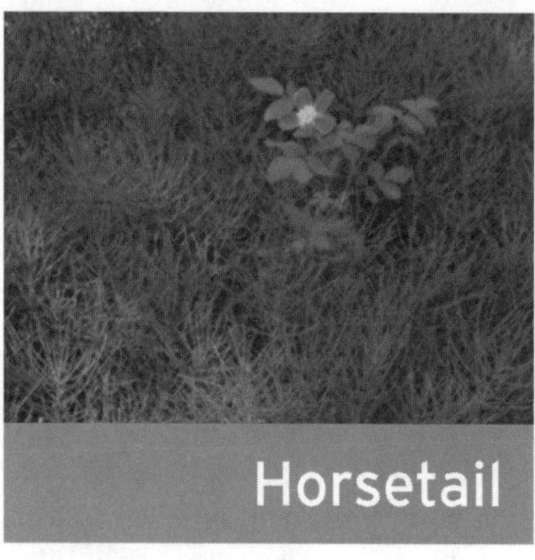

Horsetail

Equisetum arvense

Common names: Bottlebrush, Common Horsetail, Field Horsetail, Shave Grass, Shave-tail Grass.

Parts Used: Aerial parts.

Horsetail is a common plant found in the loamy soils of Europe, Asia, North Africa, and the Americas. It has long, needle-shaped leaves and small yellow fruit. This herb is prized for its silica content, over 70 percent. Silica is valuable in strengthening and repairing body tissue and enhancing the absorption of calcium.

Uses: Horsetail is an astringent especially valuable with urinary tract infection and inflammation and is an excellent clotting agent. The silica in horsetail speeds the repair of damaged tissue and improves tone and elasticity. Horsetail is also useful in the treatment of rheumatism and enlarged prostate.

Actions:
- Astringent
- Diuretic
- Vulnerary

Vaporization Temperature: 200–300°F

Warnings: Horsetail breaks down vitamin B1; therefore, long-term horsetail use should be accompanied by a vitamin B supplement. Avoid horsetail if you suffer from severe edema.

Hyssop

Hyssopus officinalis

Common names: —

Parts Used: Aerial parts.

Hyssop is a bushy evergreen with linear clusters of violet flowers. This plant proliferates southern Europe and countries throughout the Mediterranean. At one time, hyssop was regarded as a veritable "cure-all", and the Greek physician Dioscorides prescribed Hyssop in combinations with other herbs for pleurisy, asthma, and bronchial congestion.

Despite consistent benefits, this herb has grown undervalued over time and is only now becoming widely recognized once again.

Uses: The volatile oil of the Hyssop is valued for its ability to suppress spasms and stimulate the expulsion of excess gas from the body. Hyssop treats everything from chronic bronchitis to the common cold. Hyssop will strengthen the respiratory system, cool fevers, and reduce inflammation particularly in cases of asthma. The herb also calms the nervous system and is used to treat anxiety and hysteria. These nervine properties have also been used to treat mild forms of epilepsy; however, cases have been reported where certain doses of this herb's essential oil have actually exacerbated epileptic symptoms and triggered seizures. Caution for epileptics is advised.

Actions:
- Expectorant
- Diaphoretic
- Stimulant
- Pectoral
- Carminative
- Nervine
- Sedative

Vaporization Temperature: 200 – 300°F

Warnings: Epileptics should seek professional supervision before using this herb.

Kava Kava

Piper methysticum

Common names: Kava, Awa, Intoxicating Pepper, Ava Pepper.

Parts Used: Root.

Kava kava is an evergreen shrub with heart-shaped leaves that originates in the Pacific islands. Juice from the kava kava root holds great significance in the spiritual and social ceremonies of this region. Kava kava is cultivated in both the United States and Australia. Today this herb is especially popular for its slightly intoxicating effect.

Uses: Kava kava acts as both a stimulant and sedative. Its initial effect is stimulation of the nervous system, followed by a calming sensation. Feelings of euphoria have been associated with this, and the herb has a reputation as an aphrodisiac. The herb also has antiseptic properties useful in the treatment of venereal diseases and urinary infections. Kava kava may also be used to treat chronic pain, arthritis, and anxiety related disorders.

Actions:

- Stimulant
- Nervous Tonic
- Antiseptic
- Analgesic
- Sedative
- Hypnotic

Vaporization Temperature: 350 – 400°F

Warnings: Since the mid 1990s, controversy has erupted over the potential toxicity of prolonged kava kava use. Despite recent years of clinical research and data analysis, evidence remains contradictory and inconclusive. In light of this, the American Botanical Council suggests the following guidelines: avoid kava kava if suffering any liver disorder, if taking medications that adversely affect the liver, or if regularly consuming alcohol. Daily consumption of kava kava should not exceed periods of four weeks. Discontinue kava kava use at first sign of jaundice (dark urine, yellowing skin or eye tone).

Lavender

Lavandula angustifolia

Common names: English Lavender, Garden Lavender, True Lavender

Parts Used: Flowers.

Lavender is a shrubby plant with spiky green leaves and violet flowers. It is native to the western Mediterranean and is cultivated worldwide for aromatic and medicinal purposes.

Uses: Lavender is renowned for its calming and soothing properties. It is a strengthening tonic to the nervous system and a gentle relaxant. Alone and in combination with other herbs, lavender is used to relieve depression, insomnia, irritability, and headaches. It is also helpful against digestive problems and asthma.

Actions:

- Carminative
- Anti-Spasmodic
- Antidepressant
- Anti-Emetic
- Nervine
- Anti-Hydrotic

Vaporization Temperature: 200°F

Warnings: None known.

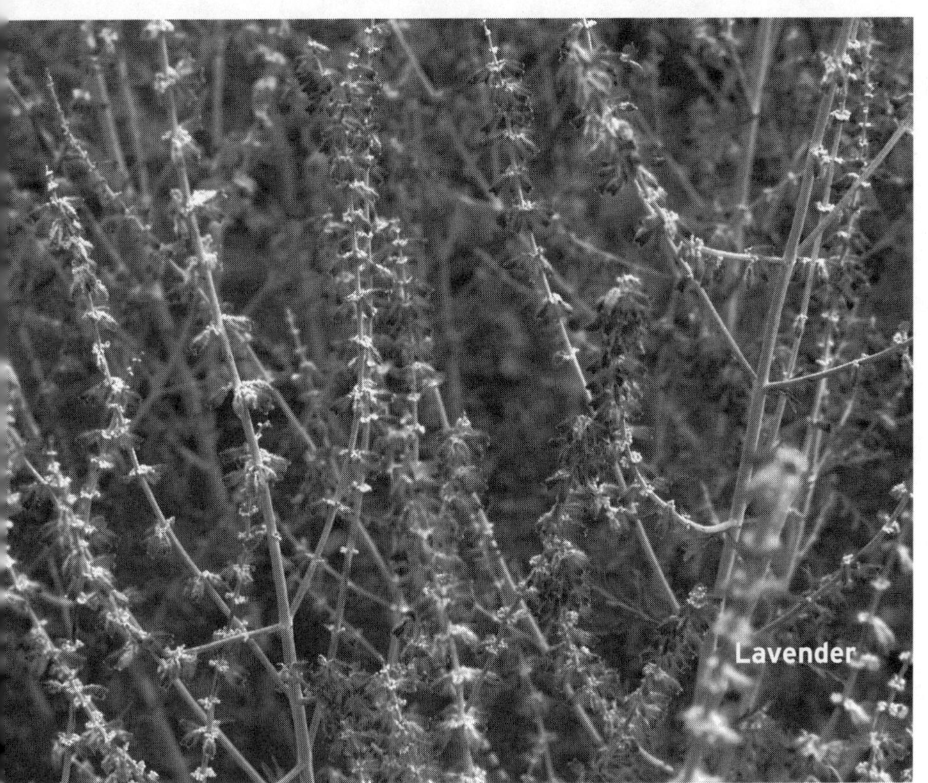

Licorice

Glycyrrhiza glabra

Common names: Liquorice, Gancao, Glycyrrhiza, Sweet Root, Yasti-madhu.

Parts Used: Root.

The licorice plant grows wild in Europe and southeast Asia. It has long slender branches and tiny spherical flowers which bloom in cone shaped umbels. Licorice is one of the most valued herbs in European herbal medicine, and its anti-inflammatory uses have been realized for thousands of years.

Uses: Licorice contains glycyrrhizic acid, which is a substance 50 times sweeter than sucrose, or table sugar. Glycyrrhizic acid is an exceptional anti-inflammatory agent helpful with such diverse conditions as asthma, mouth sores, and cirrhosis of the liver. Licorice also has a profound effect on the endocrine system and is beneficial against glandular problems such as Addison's disease. This herb also helps with digestive inflammation and joint pain.

Actions:
- Anti-Inflammatory
- Expectorant

• Demulcent
• Anti-Spasmodic
• Adrenal Agent
• Pectoral
• Mild Laxative
• Emollient

Vaporization Temperature: 350–400°F

Warnings: None known.

Marshmallow

Althaea officinalis

Common names: Marsh Mallard, Maul, Schloss Tea, Mortification Koot.

Parts Used: Root, leaves, flowers.

The mallows are a family of herbs with varying medicinal properties. In this herbal, we will address only one of the more common: the marshmallow. This erect, downy plant may grow up to seven feet in height and produces pink flowers and serrated leaves. Marshmallow originated in Europe but has naturalized to the Americas and, as its name suggests, this plant prefers mainly marshy fields and tidal zones.

Uses: The abundant mucilage of this herb affords it tremendous demulcent abilities. It is often used to soothe digestive inflammations, and bronchial ailments. It may also be used as a mild laxative and to neutralize acidic problems in the stomach.

Actions:
• Demulcent
• Diuretic
• Emollient
• Vulnerary
• Expectorant
• Anti-Catarrhal
• Pectoral

Vaporization Temperature: 200–400°F

Warnings: None known.

Meadowsweet

Spiraea ulmaria

Common names: Meadsweet, Dolloff, Queen of the Meadow, Bridewort, Lady of the Meadow.

Parts Used: Aerial parts.

Meadowsweet is native to Europe and Asia and has naturalized to the Americas. The plant may grow up to five feet tall, with thick stems and clusters of tiny yellow flowers. This fragrant wildflower was one of the most revered and sacred herbs to the Celtic Druids, who praised the herb for its spiritual qualities, but had yet to appreciate its medicinal value. Today we realize that, among other benefits, meadowsweet is rich in salicylates, which are substances which reduce inflammation and relieve pain in a method similar to aspirin. Though, unlike aspirin, salicylates do not thin the blood.

Uses: Meadowsweet is an excellent digestive aid, which is gentle enough to be used to treat diarrhea in children. Meadowsweet reduces acidity not only in the stomach, but throughout the entire body. This, along with its anti-inflammatory abilities, makes Meadowsweet an effective treatment for arthritis, rheumatism, and other ailments involving the joints.

Actions:
- Anti-Inflammatory
- Astringent
- Diuretic
- Anti-Emetic
- Aromatic

Vaporization Temperature: 200 – 300°F

Warnings: Do not use meadowsweet if allergic to aspirin.

Milk Thistle

Silybum marianum

Common names: Mary Thistle, Blessed Milk Thistle,

Parts Used: Flower heads, seeds.

Milk thistle has white marking on its leaves and bears magenta flowers in a spiky globe shape. This herb originated in the Mediterranean and has since naturalized through Europe, Australia, and the western United States. Milk thistle has a long-standing reputation as a powerful tonic for the liver, and recent scientific studies have come to support this belief.

Uses: Milk thistle is typically used to protect and strengthen the liver, especially in conditions such as hepatitis, jaundice, and cases where the liver has been damaged through alcoholism, or other external stressors. In addition, this herb is believed to increase milk production for breast-feeding mothers. Milk thistle has also been useful in the treatment of mild depression.

Actions:

- Liver Tonic
- Cholagogue
- Demulcent
- Antidepressant
- Galactagogue

Vaporization Temperature: 200 – 350°F

Warnings: None known.

Motherwort

Leonurus cardiaca

Common names: —

Parts Used: Aerial Parts.

Motherwort originated in central Asia and has naturalized to Europe and North America, where it often grows wild in woodlands, fields, and along roadsides. It has broad, jagged leaves and clusters of pink flowers. Motherwort has been valued as a heart remedy since the sixteenth century.

Uses: This herb is an excellent heart tonic, most especially conditions such as palpitations and tachycardia (extremely rapid heartbeat). It can also be used as a mild sedative and anti-spasmodic. Motherwort is an effective treatment for menstrual tension and pain as well as false labor spasms.

Actions:

- Heart Tonic
- Sedative
- Hepatic
- Nervine
- Anti-Spasmodic
- Emmenagogue

Vaporization Temperature: 200 – 300°F

Warnings: Avoid motherwort if pregnant or experiencing heavy menstrual bleeding.

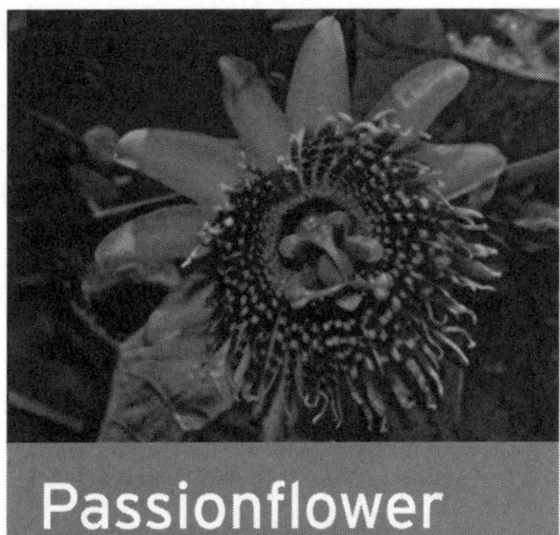

Passionflower

Passiflora incarnata

Common names: Passion Vine, Granadilla, Maracoc, Maypops.

Parts Used: Aerial parts.

Passionflower is a woody vine native to the southern United States, as well as Central and South America. Currently, it is cultivated widely throughout Europe and North America. Passionflower has been named for the flower's symbolic representation of Christ's Passion: five stamens for the five wounds.

Uses: Passionflower is a favored treatment for intransigent insomnia because it facilitates restorative sleep without a lingering narcotic heaviness. It is also valuable as an anti-spasmodic and engaged in treating disorders such as Parkinson's, epilepsy, and hysteria. Its analgesic properties allow this herb to ease conditions such as toothaches, menstrual pain, and headaches.

Actions:
- Anti-Spasmodic
- Sedative
- Hypnotic
- Nervine
- Anodyne

Vaporization Temperature: 200 – 300°F

Warnings: None known.

Peppermint

Mentha x piperita

Common names: Brandy Mint.

Parts Used: Aerial parts.

According to findings left by the ancient Greeks, Romans, and Egyptians, peppermint has been used medicinally for thousands of years. The herb was named *mentha*, for the Greek Mintha, a mythical Nymph believed to have metamorphosed into the plant. Peppermint is actually a hybrid of two mints: water mint and spearmint. Today, this herb grows wild near water sources throughout Europe and North America and is cultivated commercially worldwide.

Uses: Peppermint is most praised for its powerful carminative benefits and is widely used to relieve digestive disorders such as colic, cramps, irritable bowel, and spastic colon. As an analgesic, peppermint may be applied externally or internally to gently anesthetize the lining of the stomach and ease nausea due to motion or pregnancy. Peppermint also eases nervous tension and may soothe headaches when caused by digestive ailments. When vaporized, peppermint is an excellent treatment for nasal and bronchial congestion.

Actions:

- Carminative

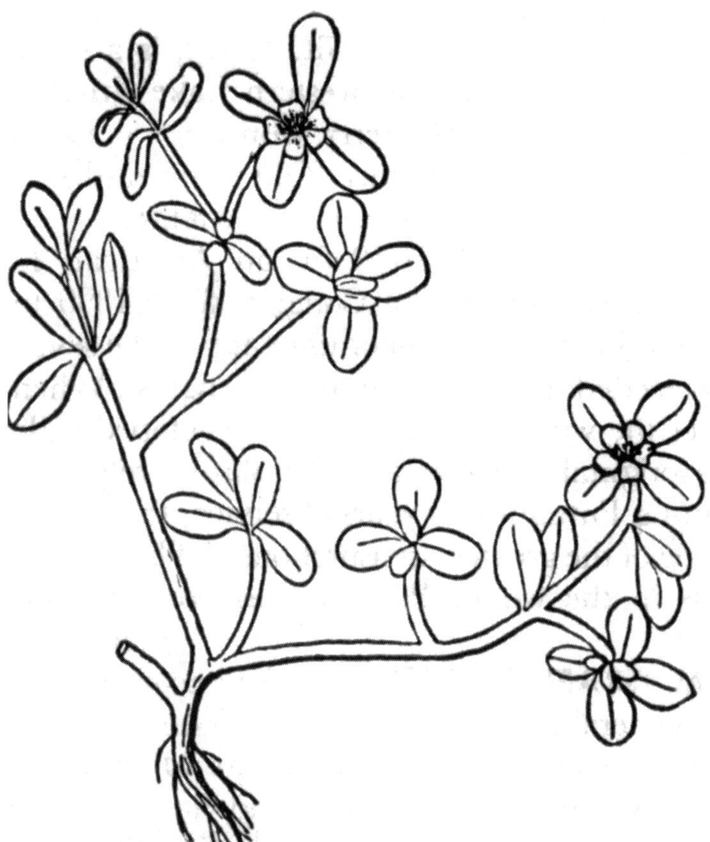

Purslane

- Rubefacient
- Aromatic
- Anti-Spasmodic
- Anti-Emetic
- Nervine
- Analgesic
- Anti-Catarrhal
- Anti-Microbial
- Emmenagogue
- Diaphoretic
- Stimulant

Vaporization Temperature: 200 – 300°F

Warnings: Do not use peppermint with children under five.

Purslane

Portulaca oleracea

Common names: Pigweed, Little Hogweed, Postelijn, Pourpier, Portulak (French), Purslane, Purslave, Pursley, Pusley.

Parts Used: Aerial parts.

Purslane has fat, tear-shaped leaves and a thick reddish stem. It originated in Europe and Asia, but is now found throughout the world. In ancient Rome, purslane had a variety of uses such as the treatment of headache, fever, and intestinal worms.

Uses: Purslane is an excellent treatment for digestive disorders and, as a diuretic, is often helpful with urinary infections. This herb is filled with antioxidant vitamins such as A, C, and E as well as the immune system booster glutsthione. Recent research has verified purslane's antibiotic properties as well.

Actions:
- Diuretic
- Anti-Pyretic
- Anti-Inflammatory
- Analgesic
- Anthelmintic
- Cholagogue

Vaporization Temperature: 200 – 300°F

Warnings: Avoid medicinal use of purslane during pregnancy.

Red Poppy

Papaver rhoeas

Common names: Corn Rose, Corn Poppy, Flores Rhoeados, Flanders Poppy, Headache.

Parts Used: Petals, seeds.

The red poppy originated in Europe and has since naturalized throughout North America. The plant may grow up to three feet tall and bears bright red flowers with a purple-black smudge at the base of each petal. Flavorful syrup is often derived from the petals and, in some areas of Germany, the seeds are used in baked goods or ground into culinary oil.

Uses: This herb contains the barest narcotic effect when compared to its cousin, the opium poppy. Still, it is used as a gentle sedative, and to soothe cough and throat irritations. When vaporized, red poppy is especially effective with respiratory congestion. The flower is also often used in teas.

Actions:

- Mild Sedative
- Expectorant
- Anti-Catarrhal

Vaporization Temperature: 200–350°F

Warnings: None known.

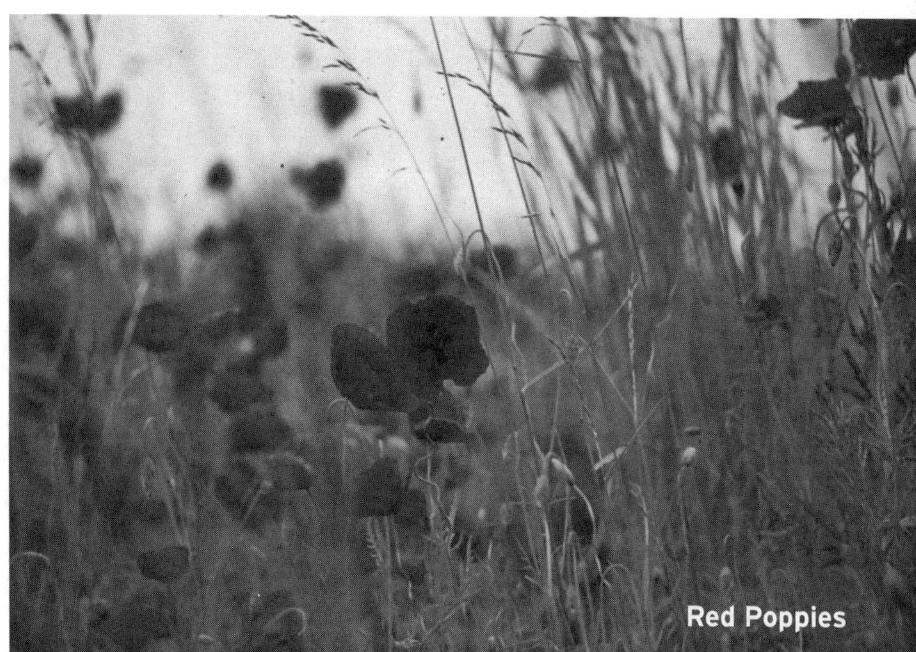

Red Poppies

Rue

Ruta graveolens

Common names: Herb-of-Grace, Herbygrass, Garden Rue.

Parts Used: Aerial parts.

Rue grows wild in the Mediterranean and is cultivated worldwide. Rue has lobe-shaped leaves and yellow and green flowers. The plant has a sharp, unpleasant odor and severely bitter taste. Rue was used in the regulation of menstruation as far back as ancient Egypt and ancient Greece.

Uses: This herb is powerfully stimulating and is often used to tone the muscles of the uterus and promote menstrual bleeding. Rue has also been used to treat intestinal worms, colic and epilepsy. Its anti-spasmodic properties aid in reducing gripping, bowel tension, and spasmodic coughs.

Actions:
- Emmenagogue
- Anti-Spasmodic
- Bitter
- Stimulant
- Rubefacient
- Abortifacient

Vaporization Temperature: 200 – 300°F

Warnings: Excess doses of rue may be toxic. To avoid skin irritation, use gloves when handling the fresh plant. Large amounts of rue may have an abortive effect. Never take rue during pregnancy.

Sage

Salvia officinalis

Common names: Sawge, Garden Sage, Red Sage, Salvia Salvatrix.

Parts Used: Leaves.

Sage is an evergreen undershrub from the Mediterranean that now thrives in cultivation throughout the world. Ancient Egyptians used this herb as a fertility drug. In addition, several species of sage are prevalent in Ayurvedic medicine, especially for the relief of gastrointestinal disorders. The curative properties of sage are evident in its botanical name. Salvia comes from the Latin *salvere,* "to save", or *salvare,* "to cure". The reputation of this herb pervaded folklore across the ages. "Why should a man die whilst Sage grows in his garden?" This Medieval saying demonstrates the esteemed reputation of the herb, as does this English proverb, "He that would live for aye / Must eat Sage in May."

Uses: Sage, widely used for its culinary spice, offers an array of therapeutic benefits. Sage may be used to aid dyspeptic conditions, relieve menstrual ailments and facilitate lactation. When vaporized, sage's astringent and antiseptic agents treat sore throat and mouth ulcers. Sage also promotes strong, healthy gums and oral cleanliness; the herb is an ingredient in most brands of toothpowder. Sage is also a helpful remedy against asthma, a powerful antioxidant, and studies are beginning to reveal sage's power against the onset of Alzheimer's disease.

Actions:

- Astringent
- Nervine
- Carminative
- Anti-Microbial
- Anti-Pyretic
- Anti-Hydrotic
- Anti-Catarrhal
- Emmenagogue
- Stimulant

Vaporization Temperature: 250–300°F

Warnings: Avoid medicinal use of sage if pregnant or epileptic.

Saint-John's-Wort

Hypericum perforatum

Common names: Hypericum, Klamathweed

Parts Used: Aerial parts.

Saint-John's-wort grows in temperate regions worldwide. Growing wild, the plant may reach three feet in height with a profusion of star-shaped yellow flowers. The subject of much superstition, "Hypericum" translates from the Greek as "over an apparition", which refers to the Medieval belief that burning this herb would ward off evil spirits in the ill.

Uses: Saint-John's-wort is widely used for disorders of the nervous system, especially chronic anxiety, sleep ailments, and depression. It should be noted that the effects of this herb on nervous disorders appear gradually and Saint-John's-wort should be taken for at least one month before determining its usefulness. In addition to the nervous system, this herb acts as a pain-reliever and sedative, and, when applied externally, as an anti-inflammatory agent.

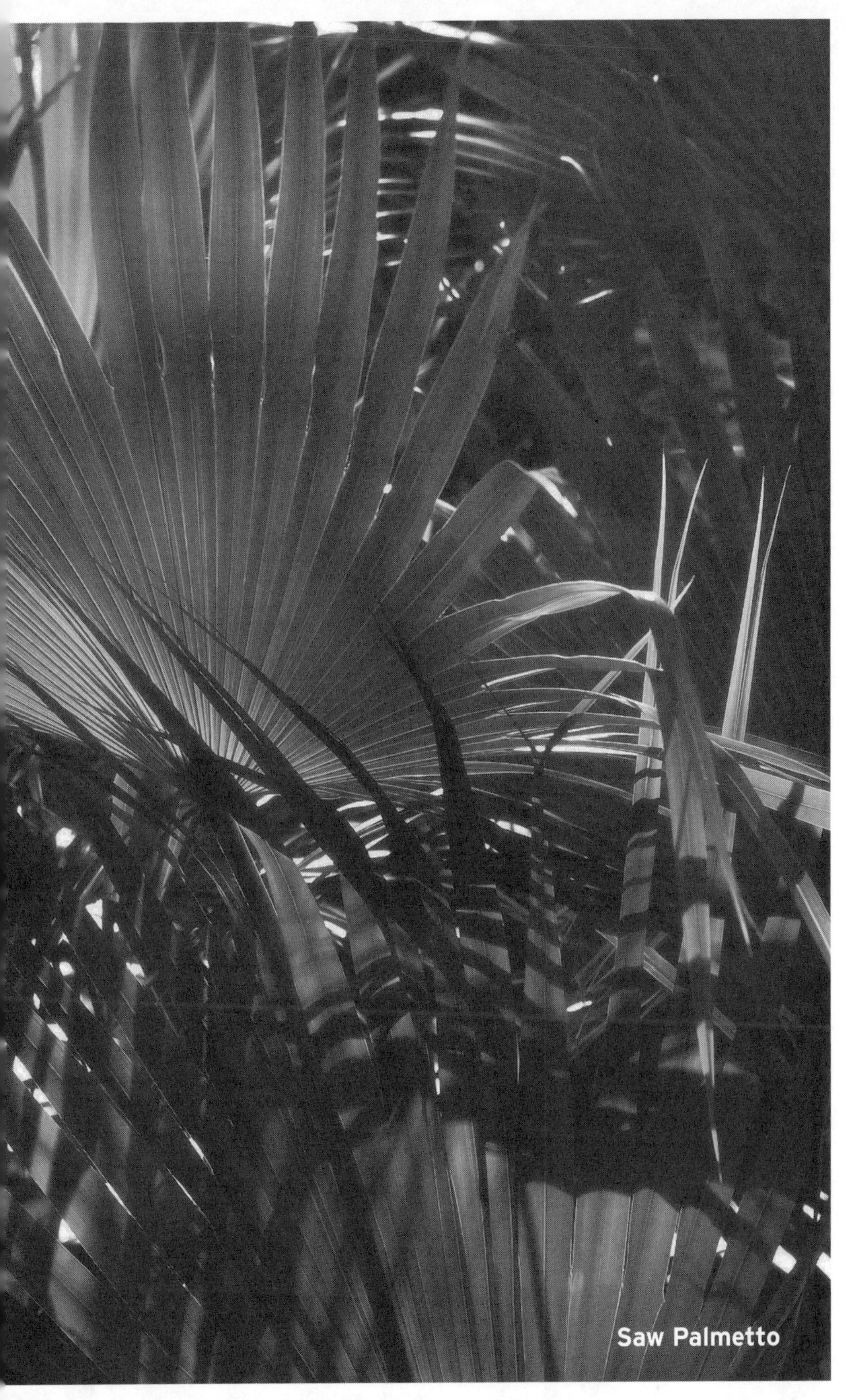
Saw Palmetto

Actions:
- Vulnerary
- Sedative
- Anti-Inflammatory
- Astringent
- Analgesic
- Expectorant

Vaporization Temperature: 200 – 300°F

Warnings: None known.

Saw Palmetto

Seronoa repens

Common names: Sabal, Sabal Serrulata.

Parts Used: Ripe fruit (berries), seeds.

Saw palmetto is a scrubby plant with long sword-like leaves a full green-blue berries that contain a strong nutty vanilla flavor. Native to North America, saw palmetto can also be found along the Atlantic coast and in the Caribbean.

Uses: Saw palmetto works as a diuretic and antiseptic for urinary tract problems. In fact, the herb has earned the nickname " plant catheter" because of its ability to shrink an enlarged prostate and tone and strengthen the bladder. Saw palmetto also has anabolic properties, allowing the herb to enhance muscle and body tissue, thereby promoting weight gain. Additionally, saw palmetto can enrich the male reproductive system, and add a boost to male hormones.

Actions:
- Anti-Inflammatory
- Anti-Spasmodic
- Diuretic
- Urinary Antiseptic
- Endocrine Agent

Vaporization Temperature: 250 – 350°F

Warnings: Avoid saw palmetto if you are pregnant, breast-feeding, or if you are taking hormone medication, or have a hormone-dependent cancer.

Sida Cordifolia

Sida Cordifolia

Common names: Sida herbacea, Sida rotundifolia, Sida althaeitolia, Bala, Bariar.

Parts Used: Root.

This perennial shrub can be found in the tropical and sub-tropical regions of India and Sri Lanka . It has long been used in Ayurvedic medicine to treat heart disease.

Uses: Today, this herb is a potent stimulant and a valuable performance booster, diaphoretic, and demulcent. It combats bronchitis, asthma and fever, cold and flu, congestion, and general edema. It may be used externally as an analgesic and anti-inflammatory agent against wounds, skin disorders, or external tumors.

Actions:
- Stimulant
- Anti-Inflammatory
- Diaphoretic
- Diuretic
- Demulcent

Vaporization Temperature: 350 – 400°F

Warnings: Sida cordifolia contains the compounds ephedrine and psuedoephedrine and the same cautions should be used as when taking Ephedra: Avoid this herb while pregnant. If you experience dizziness, severe headache, rapid heartbeat, shortness of breath, or excessive anxiety, your dose of ephedra is probably too high. If symptoms persist seek professional advice.

Thyme

Thymus vulgaris

Common names: Common Thyme, Garden Thyme.

Parts Used: Aerial parts.

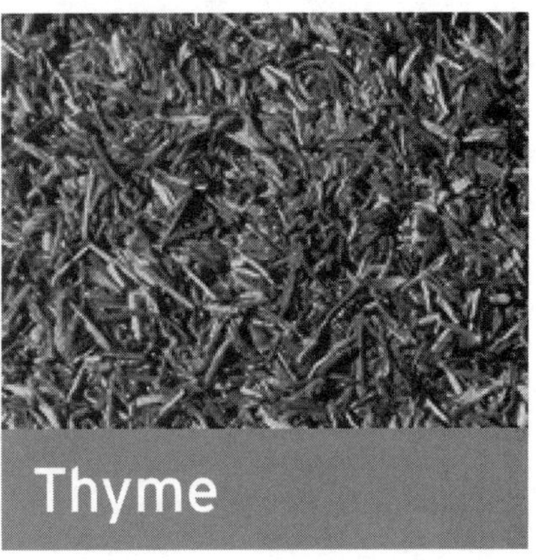

Thyme has long stalks with clusters of small pink flowers and tongue-shaped leaves. It can be found in the temperate climates of most countries. In the seventeenth century, English herbalist Nicholas Culpepper declared thyme a vigorous tonic for the lungs and superlative treatment for the then-endemic whooping cough in children.

Uses: Today, thyme is still used to benefit the respiratory system and is often used to ease asthma and hay fever, especially in children. When vaporized, thyme soothes sore throat, eases laryngitis and quells irritating cough. Externally, thyme is also used to treat infected wounds. Thyme's volatile oil is extremely antiseptic, which make it a valuable immune system booster and expectorant. Recent evidence suggests thyme is imbued with anti-aging properties and strong antioxidant powers.

Actions:
- Astringent
- Respiratory Tonic
- Carminative
- Vulnerary
- Anti-Microbial
- Anti-Spasmodic
- Anti-Catarrhal
- Expectorant
- Anthelmintic
- Antioxidant

Vaporization Temperature: 200 – 300°F

Warnings: Medicinal use of Thyme is not recommended during pregnancy.

Turmeric

Curcuma longa

Common names: Curcuma, Curcuma Rotunda, Amomum Curcuma, Indian saffron, Haldi (Hindi), Jianghuang (Chinese), Kyoo or Ukon (Japanese).

Parts Used: Rhizome.

Turmeric is native to India and southern Asia. Its bright orange flesh and spicy taste has flavored Indian cuisine for centuries. The use of turmeric for jaundice and other liver disorders dates back to ancient Chinese and Ayurvedic medicine. The cultivation of this herb has now spread throughout Africa.

Uses: Turmeric is especially effective against various skin conditions as its anti-inflammatory properties act well against arthritis, asthma, and eczema. This herb also protects and aids liver function, is an effective antioxidant, and is believed a potential preventative for those at risk for cancer. Recent clinical trials have confirmed Turmeric's ability to significantly lower cholesterol.

Actions:

- Anti-Bilious
- Anti-Inflammatory
- Antioxidant
- Anti-Bacterial
- Mild Stimulant

Vaporization Temperature: 350 – 400°F

Warnings: When taken medicinally, turmeric has been known to cause skin rashes and hypersensitivity to sunlight. Avoid turmeric if you suffer from bile duct obstruction or gallstones.

Valerian

Valeriana officinalis

Common names: Phu (Galen), All-Heal, Amantilla, Setwall, Setewale Capon's Tail.

Parts Used: Rhizome, root.

The valerian plant is native to Europe and Northern Asia and thrives in damp conditions. The valerian root has been used as a relaxant for thousands of years, dating to 1 AD when the Roman physician Dioscorides named it *Phu*, a reflection of the herbs offensive smell.

Uses: Valerian root is one of the most potent nervines available and helpful for almost any stress-related condition including anxiety, high blood pressure, and insomnia. It is often valued for producing a calming, rather than strongly sedating effect. Additionally, this herb can be beneficial as a pain reliever and anti-spasmodic.

Actions:
- Sedative
- Hypnotic
- Anti-spasmodic
- Aromatic
- Nervine
- Hypotensive
- Carminative

Vaporization Temperature: 350 – 400°F

Warnings: None known.

A Hong Kong Herbalist's Stall

Wild Yam

Dioscorea villosa

Common names: Dioscorea, Colic Root, Rheumatism Root, Wilde Yamwurzel.

Parts Used: Root and tuber (underground, bud-bearing stem).

Wild yam has long, gnarled rootstocks with many branches. It originated in North and Central America and is now cultivated in temperate climates around the world. Wild yam was widely used by the Mayans for its analgesic effects. Wild yam contains the hormone-like substance diosgenin and was used to create contraceptive medication, although the herb appears to have no contraceptive powers on its own.

Uses: Wild yam is most widely used for its potency against gynecological problems. Wild yam relaxes the uterus and eases menstruation, ovarian discomfort, and labor pain. This herb's anti-spasmodic effects are also useful to relieve intestinal cramping and overall muscle tension. Arthritis and rheumatism are also benefited from the use of wild yam.

Actions:
- Anti-Spasmodic
- Anti-Inflammatory
- Cholagogue
- Anti-Rheumatic
- Hepatic
- Anti-Bilious

Vaporization Temperature: 400°F

Warnings: None known.

Wormwood

Artemisia absinthium

Common names: Green Ginger.

Parts Used: Leaves.

Wormwood is a woody shrub with scraggly, pale green leaves. Native to Europe, this aromatic plant now grows wild in central Asia and parts of the eastern United States. As suggested by its botanical name, wormwood is an exceptionally bitter herb; *absinthium* translates to "without sweetness".

Uses: Wormwood stimulates and regulates digestion by increasing acid and bile formation in the stomach, enhancing the absorption of vital nutrients, and reducing gas

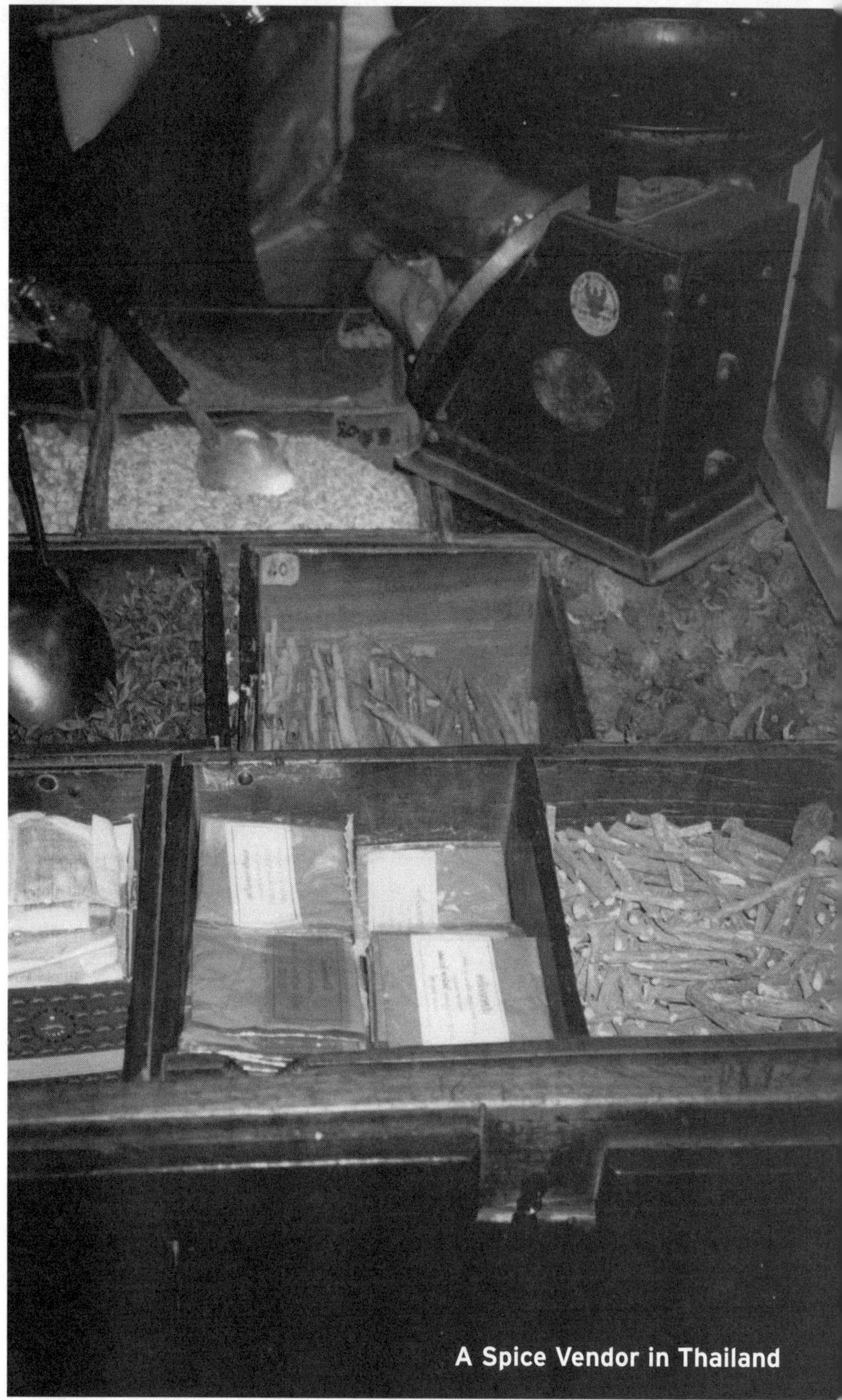

A Spice Vendor in Thailand

and bloating in the intestines. Wormwood is also a traditional remedy for eliminating worms, and promoting overall health. When topically applied, wormwood is an effective insect repellent. To avoid the intensely bitter flavor, many now vaporize this herb.

Actions:

- Bitter Tonic
- Carminative
- Emmenagogue
- Anthelmintic
- Hepatic
- Anti-Inflammatory
- Anti-Bilious
- Anti-Microbial
- Stimulant
- Mild Antidepressant

Vaporization Temperature: 200 – 300°F

Warnings: None known.

Yarrow

Achillea millefolium

Common names: Milfoil. Achillea, Millefolium, Old Man's Pepper, Soldier's Woundwort, Herbe Militaris, Thousand Weed, Nose Bleed, Carpenter's Weed. Bloodwort, Staunchweed, Sanguinary, Devil's Nettle, Devil's Plaything, Yarroway.

Parts Used: Aerial parts.

Yarrow has long been reputed for its vulnerary qualities. It was used to staunch war wounds through the Middle Ages and to stem common nosebleeds. The plant has a long, branched stem, plumes of tiny leaves, and thick umbels of white flowers. Native to Europe, yarrow now grows worldwide

Uses: When applied externally, yarrow facilitates the healing of flesh wounds. Internally, yarrow is an excellent remedy against cold and flu. It reduces fever and stimulates blood flow. Its bitter properties aid digestion and yarrow has been useful in regulating menstrual difficulties.

Actions:

- Astringent
- Digestive Tonic
- Vulnerary
- Anti-Inflammatory
- Diaphoretic

• Anti-Catarrhal
• Emmenagogue
• Hepatic
• Hypotensive
• Mild Diuretic

Vaporization Temperature: 200–300°F

Warnings: None known.

Yerba Maté

Ilex paraguariensis

Common names: Maté, Paraguay Tea, Brazilian Tea, Jesuit's Tea.

Parts Used: Leaves.

Yerba maté is an evergreen shrub with white flower clusters and spherical red fruit and is found only in the tropical regions of South America. The roasted leaves have been brewed into tea for centuries. Recently, vaporization of the herb has become highly popular.

Uses: Yerba maté is a great energy booster and bolsters stamina over longer periods than other stimulants. It is widely recognized as an effective remedy for mental and physical fatigue. In addition, this herb helps alleviate ulcers, rheumatism and similar inflammatory ailments, anemia, and mild depression. It has been known to stave off fever and, when externally applied, makes a useful poultice for skin ulcers and irritations.

Actions:
• Stimulant
• Diuretic
• Astringent
• Digestive Tonic
• Vulnerary

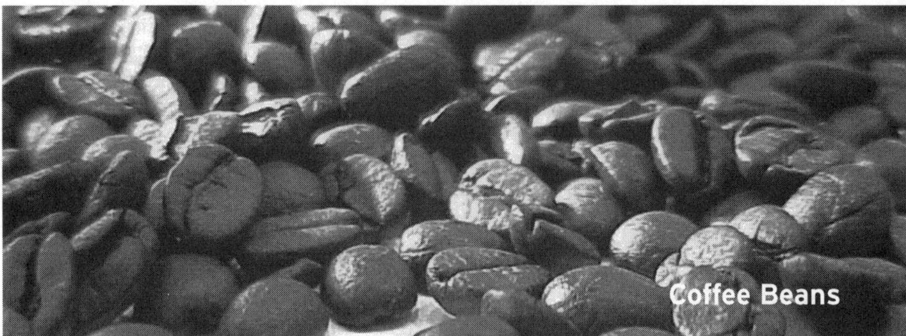
Coffee Beans

- Anti-Inflammatory
- Aromatic

Vaporization Temperature: 200 – 300°F

Warnings: None known.

HERBAL BLENDS FOR INHALATION

It is important to use a base substance when mixing a variety of plants for vaporization. The base (or carrier) substance needn't be an active ingredient in the blend. Quite often, the amount of active substances in an herbal preparation is substantially less than the amount of material needed to fill the vaporization chamber. Users will enjoy a more efficient inhalation experience if the chamber is filled; the base substances create the necessary bulk. Carriers also help perform other functions. Eucalyptus, for instance, which is one of my personal favorites, can often be used to open the breathing passageways to allow the other active elements in your blend or formula to be more easily absorbed. The carrier should be as moist or fresh as possible. Always grind the herbs and carriers that you plan to vaporize: this is crucial for the vaporization process. Hot air must pass through your herbs, and finely ground herbs will vaporize more evenly.

Here are some carrier substances I recommend and the purposes for which they are best suited:

Eucalyptus
Excellent carrier because it opens the breathing passageways. Allows easier breathing and deeper penetration of your inhaled mixture.

Mint
Nice flavor as well as an excellent carrier; it opens the breathing passageways and allows your mixture to penetrate deeper and to be breathed easily.

Sage
Stronger carrier. Excellent for smoking cessation blends.

Wild Lettuce
Lighter carrier. Excellent for smoking cessation blends.

Chamomile
Great smooth flavor. Excellent for calming effects.

Ground Guarana, Coffee or Raw Ground Chocolate
Excellent aroma. Has an invigorating stimulant effect.

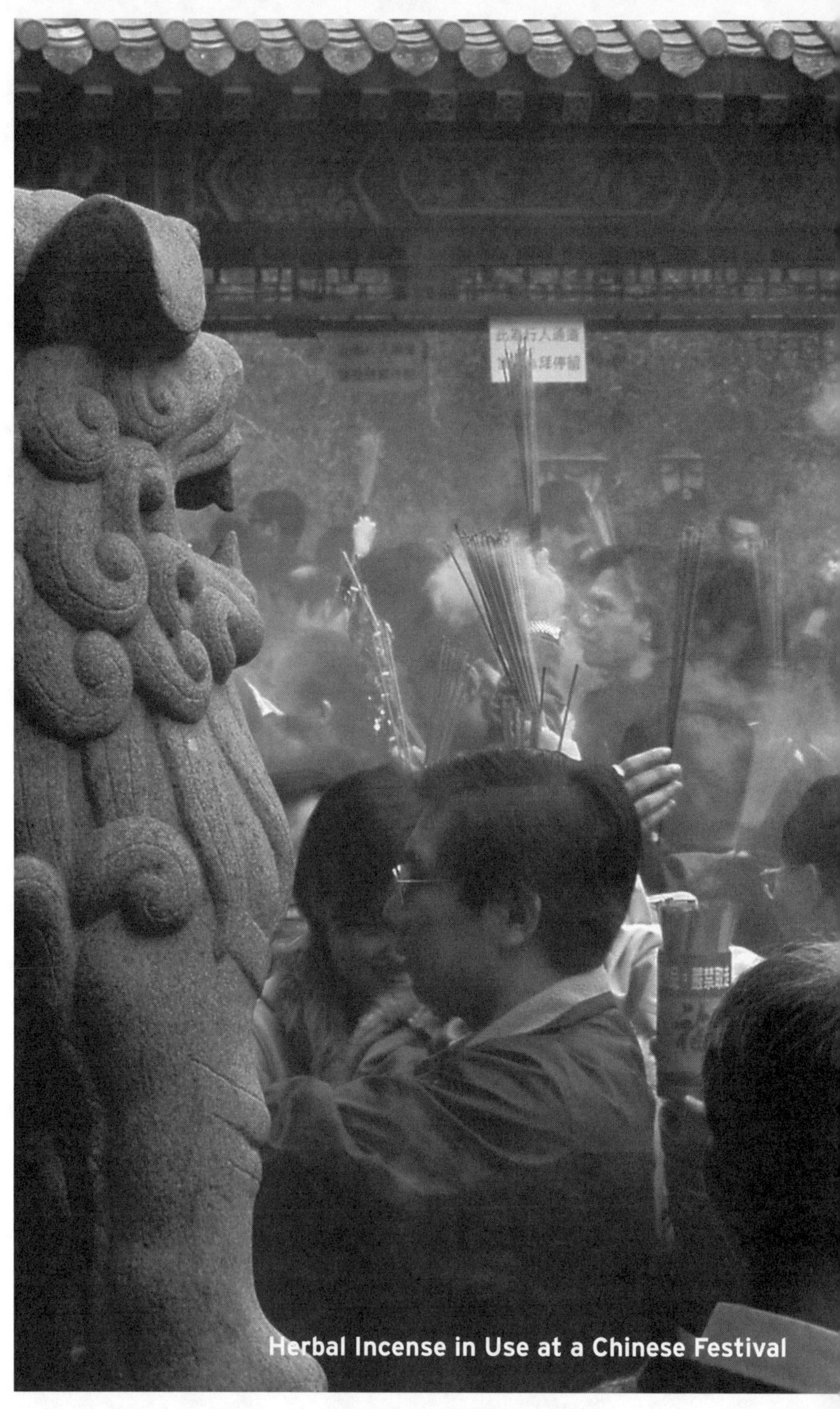

Herbal Incense in Use at a Chinese Festival

HERBAL BLENDS

Try these favorite blends for a variety of herbal enhancements!

Relaxation

3 Parts Chamomile
1 Part Wild Lettuce
1 Part Valerian
1 Part Lavender

Optional: 1-3 drops valerian extract applied to mixture.

Temperature: Pre-heat chamber to 300°F, insert materials, reduce temperature to 245°F, inhale immediately for best effects.

Invigorating / Energy

1 Part Eucalyptus
1 Part Mint
1 Part Ephedra or Sida Cordifolia
1 Part Ground Guarana of Ground Coffee

Optional : 1-3 drops of sida cordifolia or ephedra extract applied to mixture and/or 1 drop of eucalyptus essential oil.

Temperature: Pre-heat chamber to 350°F, insert materials, reduce temperature to 275°F, and inhale immediately for best effects.

Caution: This formula contains ephedrine which is derived from the ephedra or sida cordifolia plant. Those with heart, lung or other pre-existing medical conditions should consult a medical professional before trying this formula.

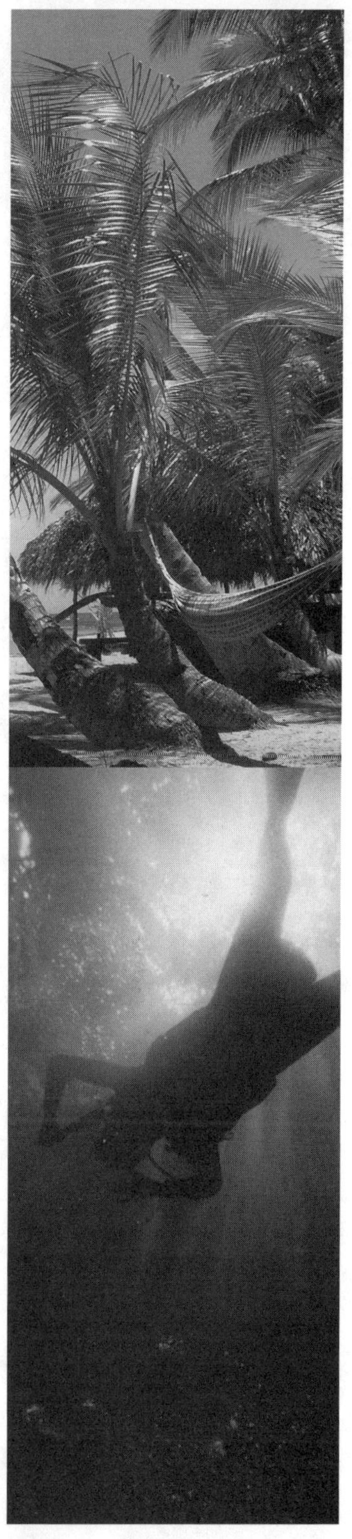

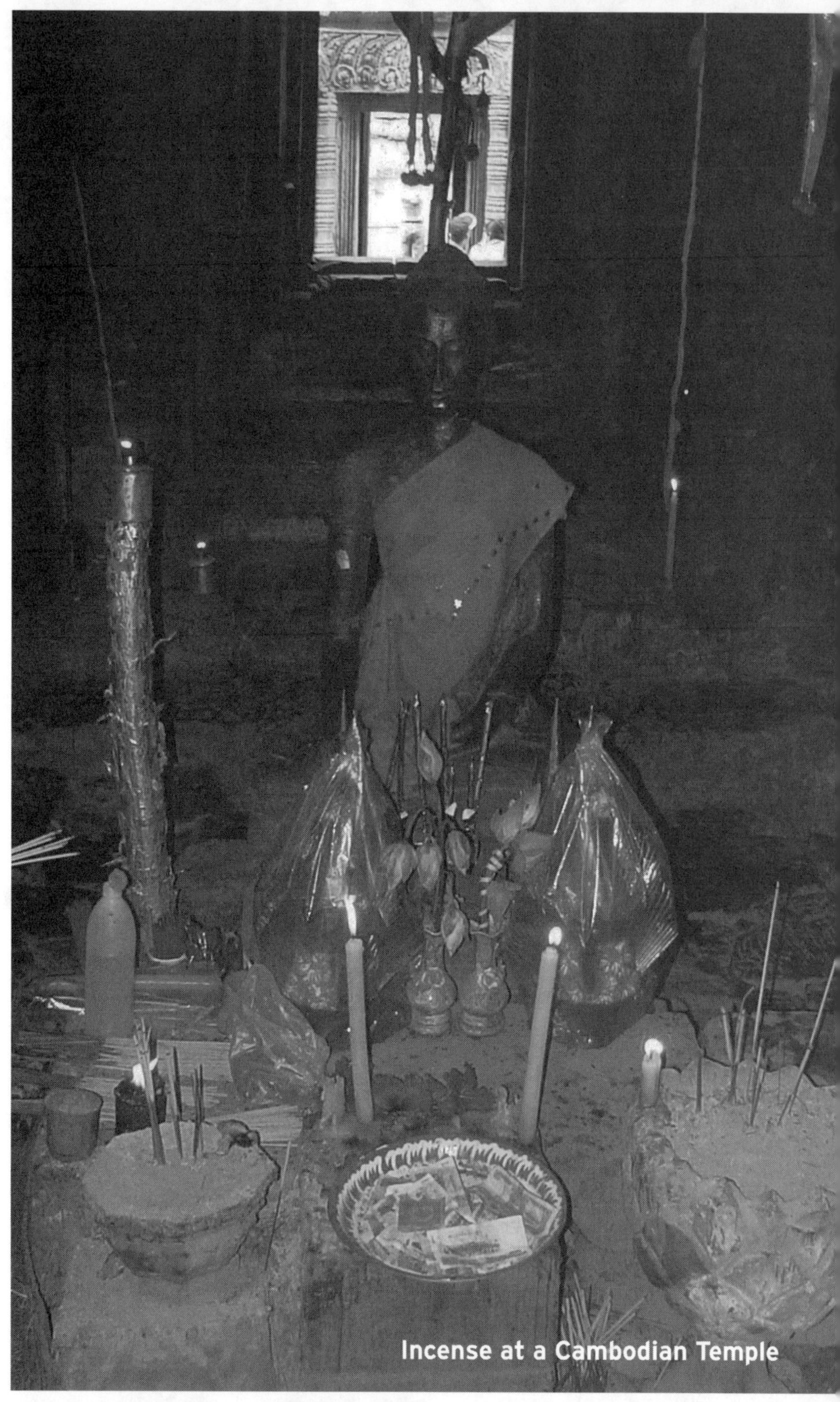

Incense at a Cambodian Temple

Mind Blend

1 Part Eucalyptus
1 Part Mint
2 Parts Ginko Biloba
2 Part Ginseng
1 Part Guarana

Optional : 1 drop Lemongrass essential oil.

Temperature: Pre-heat chamber to 350°F, insert materials, reduce temperature to 275°F, inhale immediately for best effects.

Sensual Blend For Male Vitality

1 Part Eucalyptus
1 Part Mint
1 Part Jasmine leaves
1 Part Green Tea leaves
1 Part Damiana
2 Parts Ginko Biloba
2 Part Ginseng
1 Part Guarana

Optional: 1-3 drops Sida Cordifolia or Ephedra extract applied to mixture and/or 1 drop Eucalyptus essential oil.

Temperature: Pre-heat chamber to 350°F, insert materials, reduce temperature to 275°F, inhale immediately for best effects.

Sensual Blend For Female Vitality

4 Parts Damiana
1 Part Eucalyptus
1 Part Mint
1 Part Lavender
1 Part Jasmine leaves
1 Part Green Tea leaves
2 Parts Ginko Biloba
2 Part Ginseng
1 Part Guarana

Optional: For a very special aphrodisiac add one

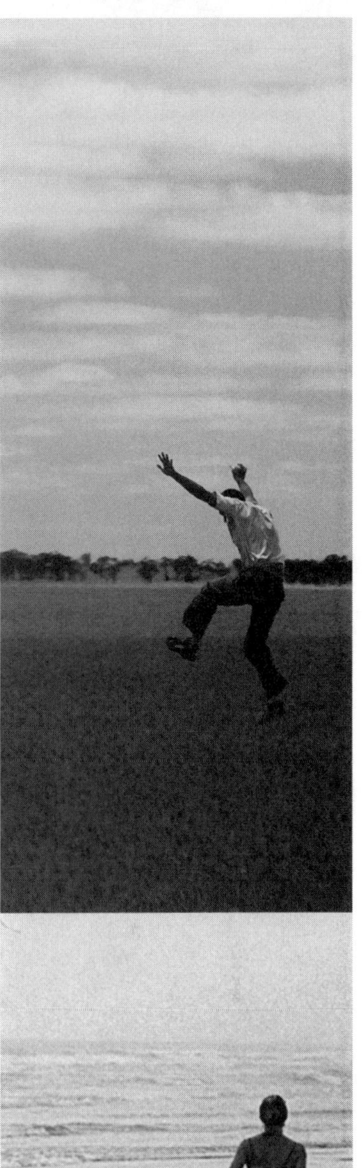

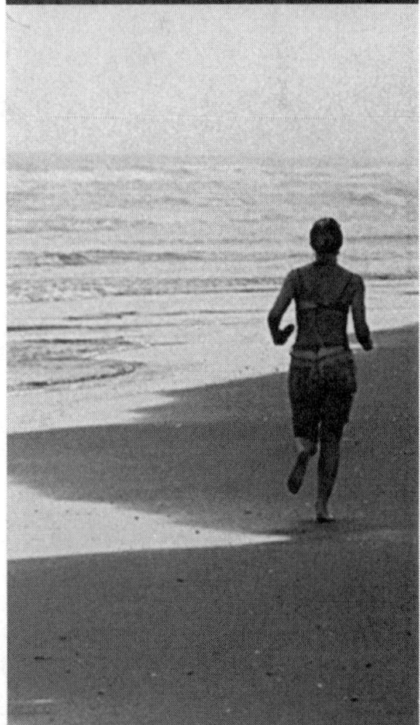

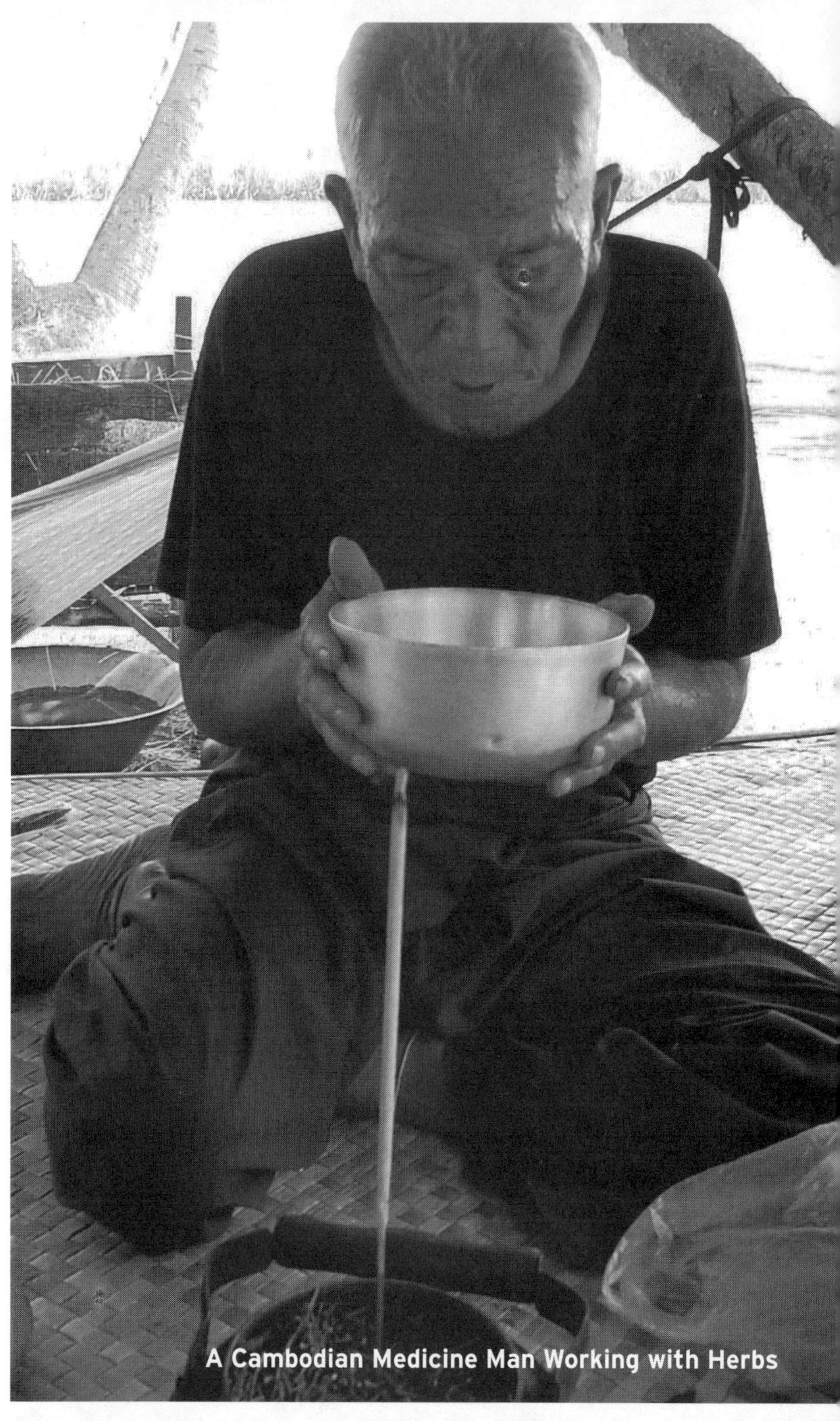
A Cambodian Medicine Man Working with Herbs

part narcissist leaves and/or one part gardena leaves. Chocolate or ground vanilla beans also make for an excellent addition.

Optional: 1-3 drops Sida Cordifolia or Ephedra extract applied to mixture and/or 1 drop of Eucalyptus essential oil.

Temperature: Pre-heat chamber to 350°F, insert materials, reduce temperature to 275°F, inhale immediately for best effects.

MORE HERBAL BLENDS

Air Fresheners (Not for direct inhalation! For ambient aromatherapy only.)
20 Parts Rosemary, 8 Parts Grapefruit, 4 Parts Peppermint, 2 Parts Spearmint.
Or try this:
20 Parts Lime, 14 Parts Bergamot, 4 Parts Ylang Ylang, 2 Parts Rose.

Asthma / Anti-spasmodic:
6 Parts Lavender, 2 Parts Hyssop, 2 Parts Marjoram

Balance and Harmony:
Equal Parts Sandalwood, Musk, Bergamot, and Lemon.

Bronchitis:
4 Parts Sandalwood, 3 Parts Eucalyptus, 3 Parts Bergamot.

Cough:
3 Parts Lavender, 2 Parts Thyme, 2 Parts Eucalyptus.
Or try this:
3 Parts Frankincense, 3 Parts Eucalyptus, 2 Parts Hyssop.

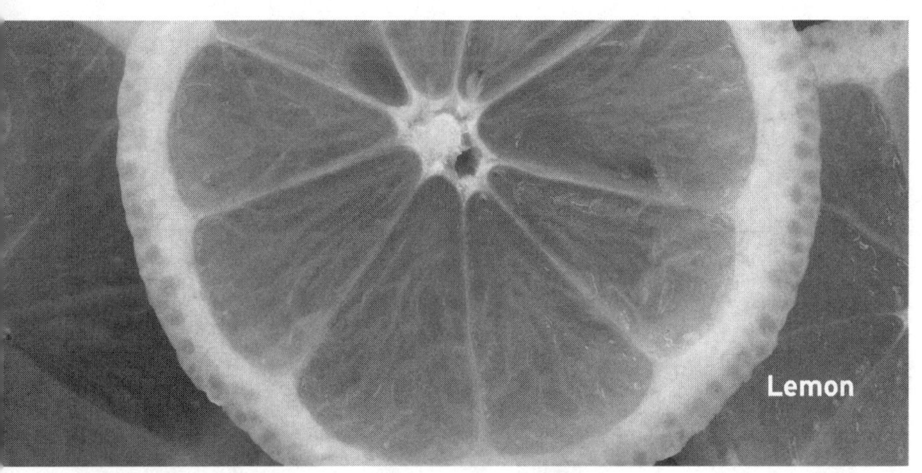
Lemon

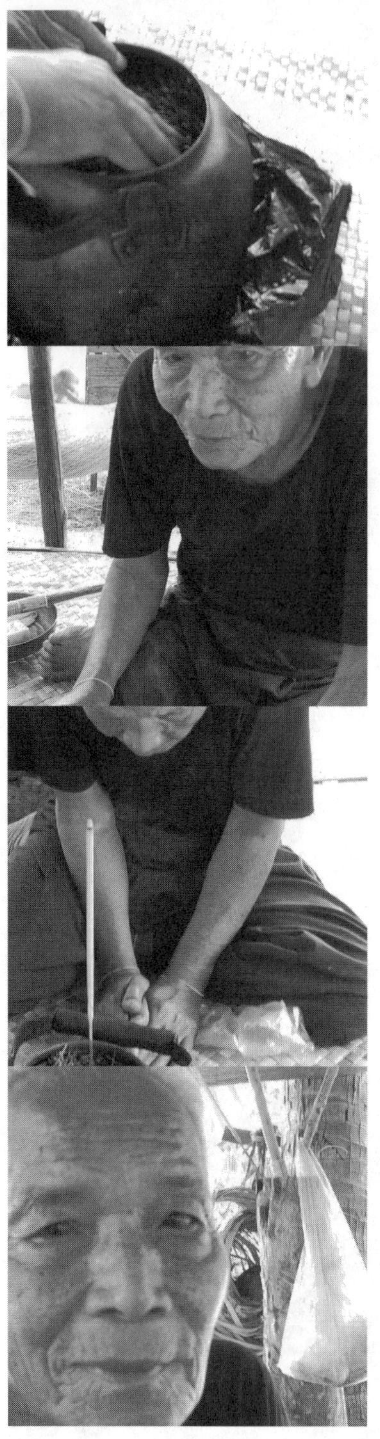

Creativity Boost:
Equal Parts Peppermint, Orange, and Rosemary.

Deodorizer:
6 Parts Bergamot, 2 Parts Lemon, 1 Parts Eucalyptus.

Detoxifying:
Equal Parts Geranium, Rosemary, and Juniper.

Dream Enhancement:
8 Parts Lavender, 8 Parts Marjoram, 3 Parts Lemon.

Headache:
9 Parts Chamomile, 8 Parts Lavender, 8 Parts Geranium.
Or try this:
6 Parts Lavender, 4 Parts Marjoram, 2 Parts Peppermint.

Head Cold / Congestion:
7 Parts Eucalyptus, 2 Parts Basil, 1 Part Peppermint.

Influenza / Cold with Fever:
7 Parts Eucalyptus, 3 Parts Camphor.

Insomnia:
3 Parts Rose, 3 Parts Sage, 3 Parts Chamomile, 2 Parts Valerian.
Or try this:
5 Parts Geranium, 4 Parts Lavender, 3 Parts Sandalwood, and 2 Parts each of Chamomile and Lemongrass.

Meditation:
8 Parts Sandalwood, 2 Parts Rosewood.

Mental Boost / Concentration:
8 Parts Ylang Ylang, 8 Parts Rosemary, 4 Parts Basil.

Painful Menstruation:
Equal Parts Lavender, Peppermint, Nutmeg, and Cypress.

Premenstrual Cramps:
Equal Parts Sage, Jasmine, and Lavender.

Relaxation:
Equal Parts Lavender, Orange, and Cedarwood.
Or try this:
Equal Parts Bergamot, Melissa, Frankincense, and Sandalwood.

Sensuality:
10 Parts Rose, 10 Parts Magnolia, 8 Parts Lemon, 2 Parts Ylang Ylang.
Or try this:
10 Parts Ylang Ylang, 10 Parts Sage, 8 Parts Sandalwood, 6 Parts Frankincense, and 4 Parts Jasmine.

Sore Throat:
3 Parts Lavender, 2 Parts Chamomile, 1 Part Thyme.

Spicy Holiday Scent:
8 Parts Cinnamon, 6 Parts Nutmeg, 6 Parts Clove, 4 Parts Frankincense, 3 Parts Orange.

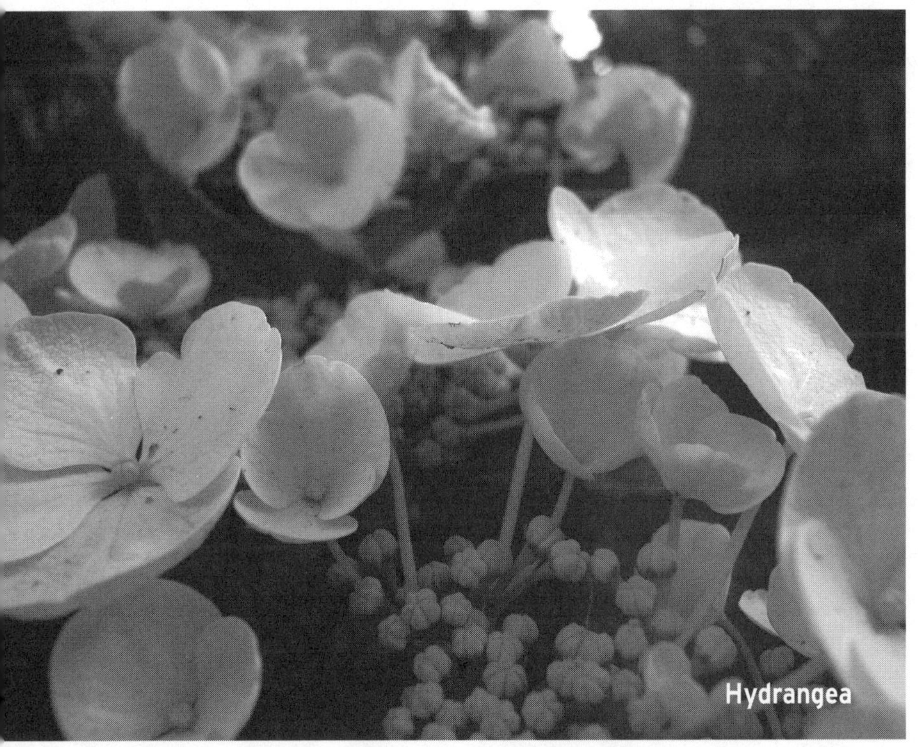

Hydrangea

Stress:
10 Parts Neroli, 7 Parts Rosemary, 8 Drops Lavender.

Uplifting:
5 Parts Lemongrass, 5 Parts Geranium, 3 Parts Sweet Basil, 2 Parts Lime.

Wintertime Refresher:
10 Parts Frankincense, 10 Parts Lemon, 7 Parts Eucalyptus, 4 Parts Thyme.

Vitality:
8 Parts Peppermint, 7 Parts Rosemary, 5 Parts Orange, 3 Parts Grapefruit, 3 Parts Lemongrass.

See the author's website, www.opill.com, for more blends.

ADDITIONAL HERBS

Echinacea
Gravel Root
Hydrangea
Elde
Lobelia
Gentian
Cramp Bark
Lady's Slipper
Rhubarb Root
Cascara Segrada
Blue Flag
Elecampane
Myrrh
Skullcap
Alfalfa
Slippery Elm
Coltsfoot
Hops
Elecampane
Sassafras

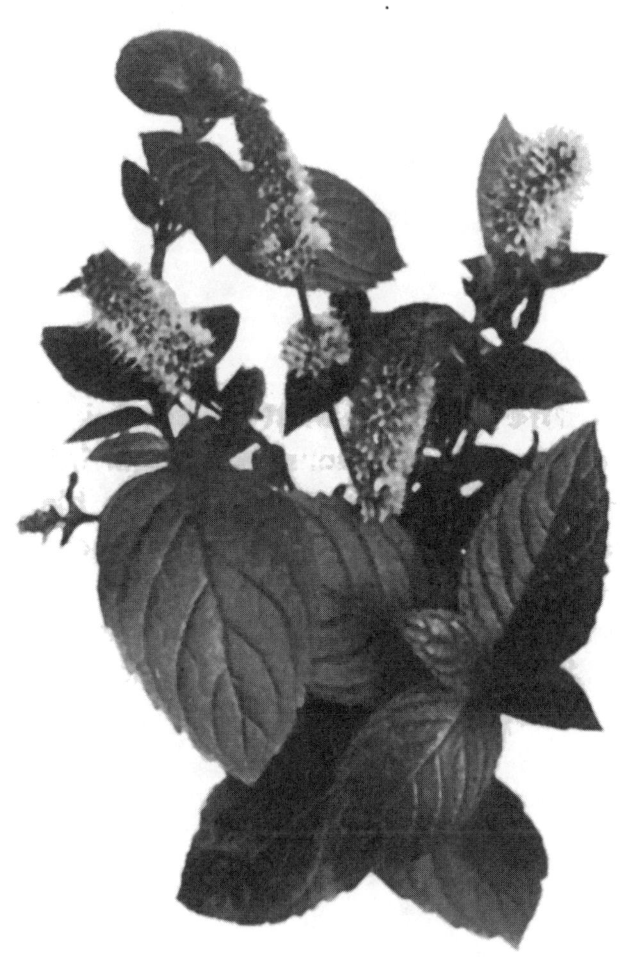

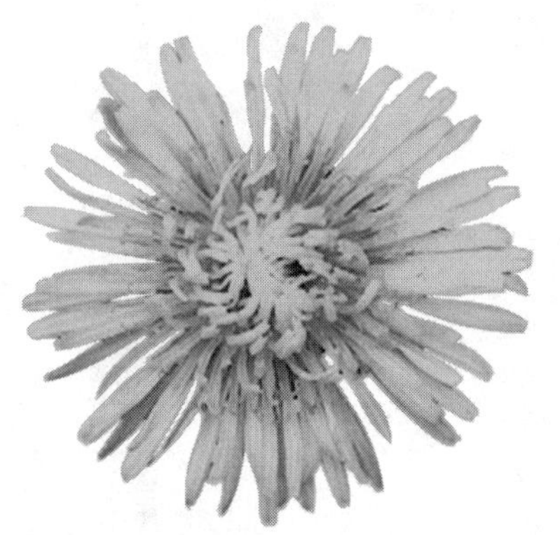

Afterword

No single book can provide you with all the information you will require on any science. Within the pages of this book you should find all of the necessary information to start you on the path to unlocking the secrets and many applications of digital vaporization. You can also find much useful information on herbs, aromatherapy and vaporization through other sources.

A final note: One of the unsung heroes of aromatherapy and vaporization was Nostradamus. The sixteenth-century French astrologer and physician, whose real name was Michel de Nostredame, is reputed to have effected remarkable cures during outbreaks of the plague in France using primitive systems of aromatherapy and vaporization. His rhymed prophecies gained him the favor of the French court but were often enshrouded in secret code to prevent from offending the powers that be.

You don't have to go too far to know that much of what Nostradamus wrote was in code. You don't have to go too far to find Michel's secret. Actually it is all around you. Like a fisherman's net, his secret can be found world wide. Don't let negative forces cast a web on Michel's secret. An 'open mind' is the key.

Notes

1 The MacGill Molson Medical Informatics as posted on HealthLink USA, 2002.

2 The World Health Organization. "In Tobacco or Health: A Global Status Report". Geneva, 1997: 43-48. Posted Healthlink USA, 2002.

3 McBride. "The health consequences of smoking: Cardiovascular disease". *The Medical Clinics of North America*, 1992; 76(2):333-353. The MacGill Molson Medical Informatics as posted on HealthLink USA, 2002.

4 National Cancer Institute, 2002.

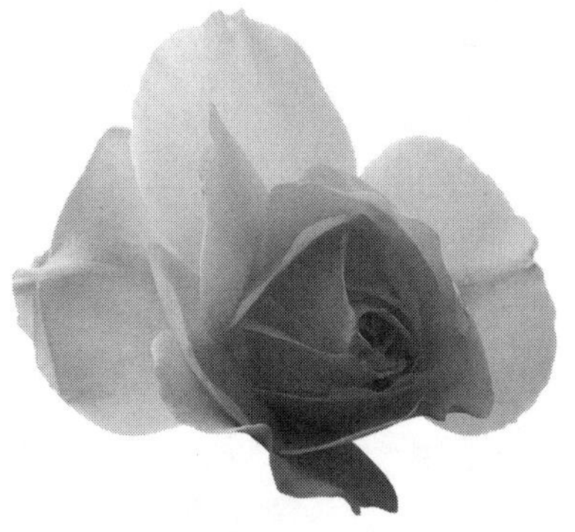

Recommended Resources

SMOKING CESSATION

American Cancer Society
1-800-227-2345
www.cancer.org

American Lung Association
61 Broadway, 6th Floor
NY, NY 10006
1-800-586-4872
www.lungusa.org

American Heart Association
National Center
7272 Greenville Avenue
Dallas, TX 75231
214-373-6300
www.amheart.org

Nicotine Anonymous
419 Main Street, PMB# 370
Huntington Beach, CA 92648
1-800-642-0666
www.nicotine-anonymous.org

National Cancer Institute
NCI Public Inquiries Office
Suite 3036A
6116 Executive Boulevard, MSC8322
Bethesda, MD 20892-8322
1-800-422-6237
www.cancernet.nci.nih.gov

www.quitnet.com

www.kickbutt.com

www.drquit.com

www.tobacco.org

www.drnicfree.com

HERBOLOGY

American Association of Naturopathic Physicians (AANP)
8201 Greensboro Drive, Suite 300
McLean, VA 22102
(877) 969-2267
www.naturopathic.org

American Botanical Council
P.O. Box 144345
Austin, Texas 78714-4345
(512) 926-4900 / (800) 373-7105
www.herbalgram.org

American Herbalist Guild
1931 Gaddis Road
Canton, GA 30115
(770) 751-6021
http://www.americanherbalistsguild.com/

The American Herb Association
Box 1673
Nevada City, CA 95949
(530) 265-9552
http://www.ahaherb.com/

American Herbalists' Guild
1931 Gaddis Road
Canton, GA 30115
(770) 751-6021
www.americanherbalistsguild.com

Council for Complimentary and Alternative Medicine (UK)
206-8 Latimer Road
London W10 6RE

The Herb Society of America, Inc.
9019 Kirkland Chardon Road
Mentor, Ohio 44094
(216) 256-0514
www.herbsociety.org

National Institute of Medicinal Herbalists (UK)
56 Longbrook Street
Exeter EX4 6AH
www.nimh.org.uk

National Association for Holistic Aromatherapy
4509 Interlake Ave N., #233
Seattle, WA 98103-6773
888-ASK-NAHA *or* (206) 547-2164
www.naha.org

The School of Phytotherapy (UK)
Bucksteep Manor
Bodle Street Green
East Sussex BN277 4RJ
tel: 44-1323-833812

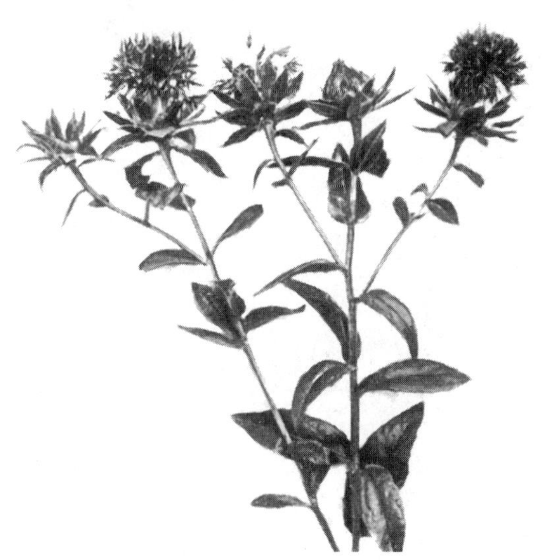

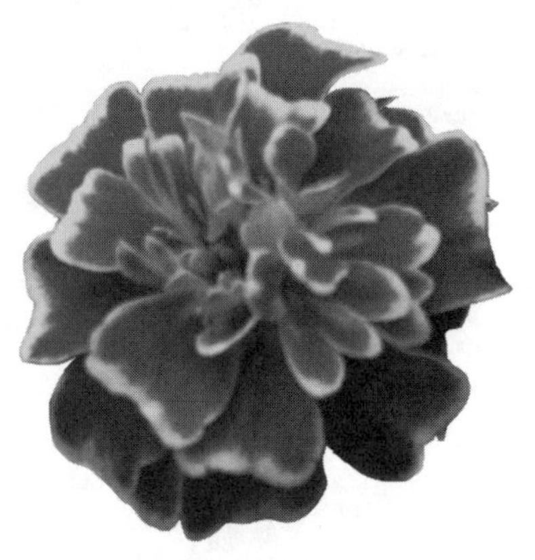

Bibliography

Aftel, Mandy. *Essence and Alchemy: A Book of Perfume.* New York, New York: North Point Press, 2001.

American Botanical Council. Herbal Medicine: Expanded Commission E Monographs. http://www.herbalgram.org/browse.php/herbal_medicine_online. (Assessed May, 2002.)

Andoh, Anthony. *The Science and Romance of Selected Herbs Used in Medicine and Religious Ceremony.* San Francisco California: North Shale Institute Education and Research Group, 1991.

Andrews, Steve. *Herbs of the Northern Shaman: A Guide to Mind-Altering Plants of the Northern Hemisphere.* Port Townsend, Washington: Loompanics Unlimited, 2000.

Angier, Bradford. *Field Guide to Medicinal Wild Plants.* Harrisburg, Pennsylvania: Stackpole Books, 1978.

Balch, Phyllis A. *Prescription for Herbal Healing.* New York, New York: Penguin Putnam, 2002.

Borgerding, M. F., and W.S. Rickert. *Summary of Scientific facts Regarding Tobacco Heating Eclipse Cigarettes.* RJ Reynolds Tobacco Company, April 2000. http://new.eclipsescience.com/results/default.html. (Assessed July 2002).

Borio, Gene. "Tobacco Timeline." Tobacco BBS, (1993 – 2001.) http://www.tobacco.org/History/Tobacco_History.html. (Assessed July 2002).

BBCi, "Medicine Through Time." http://www.washingtonpost.com/wp-srv/aponline/20011105/aponline194356_000.htm (Assessed June, 2002.)

Balz, Rodolphe. *The Healing Power of Essential Oils.* Delhi, India: Motilal Banarsidass Publishers, 1999.

Brown, Deni. *The Herb Society of America Encyclopedia of Herbs and Their Uses.* New York, New York: Dorling Kindersley Publishing, 1995.

Chavallier, Andrew. *Natural Health Encyclopedia of Herbal Medicine.* New York, New York: Doris Kindersley Publishing, 2000.

Cichoke, Anthony J. *Secrets of Native American Herbal Remedies.* New York, New York: Penguin Putnam, Inc., 2001.

Clymer, R. Swinburne. *The Medicines of Nature: The Thomsonian System.* Quakertown, Pennsylvania: The Humanitarian Society, 1926.

Coon, Nelson. *Using Plants for Healing. Emmaus,* Pennsylvania: Rodale Press, 1979.

Cunningham, Scott. *Magical Aromatherapy: The Power of Scent.* St. Paul, Minnesota: Llewellyn Publications, 1999.

DeMatteis, Bob. *From Patent to Profit: Secrets and Strategies for the Successful Inventor*. Garden City Park, New York: Avery Publishing Group, 1998.

Duke, James A. *Anti-Aging Prescriptions*. Emmaus, Pennsylvania: Rodale Press, 2001.

Duke, James A. *The Green Pharmacy*. Emmaus, Pennsylvania: Rodale Press, 1997.

De Luca, Diana. *Botanica Erotica: Arousing Body, Mind, and Spirit*. Rochester, Vermont: Healing Arts Press, 1998.

Fiore MC, Ed. *Cigarette Smoking: A Clinical Guide to Assessment and Treatment*. Philadelphia, PA: WB Saunders Co; 1992: 305-331, Medical Clinics of North America.

Fisher, Kathleen. *Herbal Remedies*. Emmaus, Pennsylvania: Rodale Press, 1999.

Fulder, Stephen. *The Ginseng Book*. Garden City Park, New York: Avery Publishing Group,1996.

Glantz, Stanton, et al. *The Cigarette Papers*. San Francisco, California: University of California Press, 1996.

Grieve, M. A *Modern Herbal*. New York, New York: Dover Publications, 1971.

Groleau, Rick. "On Fire." PBS NOVA Online. October 2, 2001. http://www.pbs.org/wgbh/nova/cigarette/onfire.html. (Assessed June, 2002.)

Herbworx International. Herbal Actions, Indications, Monographs. http://www.phytotherapies.org/index.cfm. (Assessed June, 2002.)

Hilts, Philip J. Smokescreen: *The Truth Behind the Tobacco Industry Coverup*. Reading, Massachusetts: Addison-Wesley, 1996.

Hoffman, David. *The Complete Illustrated Holistic Herbal*. Shaftesbury, Dorset, UK: Element Books, 1999.

Hylton, William H., and Claire Kowalchik, eds. *Rodale's Illustrated Encyclopedia of Herbs*. Emmaus, Pennsylvania: Rodale Press, 1987.

Washington, D.C.: National Academy of Sciences, 1999.

Krok, Lexi. "Anatomy of a Cigarette." PBS NOVA Online. October 2, 2001. http://www.pbs.org/wgbh/nova/cigarette/anatomy.html. (Assessed June 2002.)

Lust, John. *The Herb Book*. New York, New York: Bantam Books, 1974.

Mabey, Richard. *The New Age Herbalist*. New York, New York: Macmillan Publishing Company, 1988.

Metzner, Ralph. *Green Psychology: Transforming Our Relationship to the Earth*. Rochester, Vermont: Oak Street Press, 1999.

Molony, David. *The American Association of Oriental Medicine's Complete Guide to Chinese Herbal Medicine*. New York, New York: Berkley Books, 1998.

The National Center for the Preservation of Medicinal Herbs. "History of Herbalism." NCPMH. 1998. http: //www.ncpmh.org/history.html. (Assessed May, 2002.)

Parker-Pop, Tara. *Cigarettes: Anatomy of an Industry from Seed to Smoke*. New York, New York: The New Press, 2001.

Purvis, Andrew. "Ginko." *The Guardian*. November 22, 2001. http://education.guardian.co.uk/Print/0,3858,4304452,00.html (June, 2002.)

RJ Reynolds Tobacco Company. *Summary of Scientific facts Regarding Tobacco Heating Eclipse Cigarettes*.

Schreiner, Bruce. "B&W Test-Markets New Cigarette." http://www.washingtonpost.com/wp-srv/aponline/20011105/aponline194356_000.htm. November 15, 2001.

Samet, Jonathan, and Marrita S. Jaakkola, eds. "Environmental Tobacco Smoke: Risk Assessment". *Environmental Health Perspectives*, Vol.107,No. 4, April 1999.

Schwartz-Bloom, Michelle, and Gayle Gross de Núñez. "The Dope on Nicotine." PBS NOVA Online. October 2, 2001. http://www.pbs.org/wgbh/nova/cigarette/nicotine.html (Assessed June, 2002.)

Spinella, Marcello. *The Psychopharmacology of Herbal Medicine. Cambridge*. Massachusetts: The MIT Press, 2001.

Tisserand, Robert T. *The Art of Aromatherapy: The Healing and Beautifying Properties of the Essential Oils of Flowers and Herbs*. Rochester, Vermont: Healing Arts Press, 1977.

University Of Virginia Health Systems. "A Brief History of Herbalism." UVA Health Sciences Library: Historical Collections & Services. June, 1997. http://hsc.virginia.edu/hs-library/historical/herb/intro.html. (Assessed May, 2002.)

Walters, Clare. *Aromatherapy: A Basic Guide*. New York, New York: Barnes & Noble Books, 1998,

Wicke, Roger. "A world history of herbology and herbalism: oppressed arts." The Rocky Mountain Herbal Institute Online. January, 1998. http://www.rmhiherbal.org/a/f.ahr1.hist.html#abstract. (Assessed June, 2002.)

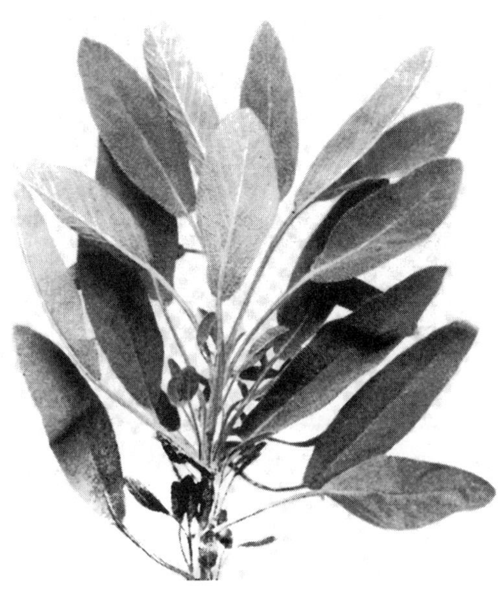

Glossary

Alveoli
Tiny, capillary-rich air sacs in the lungs where oxygen may enter the blood stream.

Alternative "Blood cleansers"
Herbs which remove toxins, restore vitality and strengthen overall bodily function and whose benefits accrue gradually.

Analgesic / Anodyne
Painkillers. An analgesic is a stronger remedy for pain; however. an anodyne may contribute an anesthetic effect as well and can be used to induce an unconscious state.

Anesthetic
A numbing agent. Anesthetics cause loss of sensation without the loss of consciousness. Many anesthetics are derviced from the coco plant (*Erythroxylum coca*).

Anthelmintic (Vermicide / Vermifuge)
An herb or medicine with properties that kill or damage intestinal worms.

Anti-Bilious
These herbs remove excess bile from the body and may be useful in treating jaundice or biliary conditions.

Antibiotic
Herb or medicine that destroys or inhibits the growth of bacteria, viruses, and other microorganisms.

Anti-Catarrhal
An herb or medicine with properties that counteract the formation and inflammation of mucus, especially in the nose and throat.

Anti-Emetic
An herb or medicine with properties that suppress or prevent nausea and vomiting.

Anti-Hydrotic
Having an inhibitory action on the secretion of sweat.

Anti-Inflammatory
An herb or medicine with properties that reduce inflammation.

Anti-Lithic
An herb or medicine with properties that dissolve and prevent further formation of urinary or biliary stones.

Anti-Microbial
An herb or medicine with properties that destroy or inhibit the growth of destructive microorganisms.

Anti-Pyretic (Febrifuge)
An herb or medicine with properties that are "cooling" herbs used in fever reduction

Antiseptic
An herb or medicine with properties which fight infection by suppressing and preventing the growth of microbes and bacteria

Antioxidant
An herb or medicine with properties that prevent or delay the damaging oxidization of the body's cells..

Anti-Spasmodic
Anti-spasmodic herbs prevent or ease muscle spasms and cramps.

Aromatic
An herb or medicine that emits a strong, pleasant, often stimulating fragrance.

Aromatherapy
The use of natural fragrance, such as essential plant oils, to affect mood and promote health and well being.

Aspirin
Analgesic derived from the Meadowsweet plant (*Filipendula ulmaria*).

Astringent
An herb or medicine that contracts tissues to reduce secretions.

Bitter
An herb or medicine with a bitter, even unpleasant flavor that stimulates the digestive system.

Caliph
A leader of an Islamic polity, regarded as a successor of Muhammad.

"Cancer By The Carton"
A landmark Reader's Digest Article published in 1952 and detailing the dangers of smoking for essentially the first time.

Carminative
Herbs with rich volatile oils that stimulate digestion and promote the expulsion of excess gas

Cassolette
A box, or vase, with a perforated cover to emit perfumes, carried by ancient physicians to ward against disease.

Ch'i
Traditional Chinese word representing "inner energy" and life force.

Cholagogue
An herb or medicine that aids with problems of the gall bladder by stimulating its secretion of bile.

Cytostatic
An herb or medicine that inhibits or suppresses cellular growth and multiplication.

Denaturization
The act of changing the inherent nature or qualities of an object. Matter often becomes denatured through combustion.

Demulcent
A soothing medicine or herb that soothes, heals, and protects inflamed tissue, especially of the digestive tract.

Diaphoretic
An herb or medicine with properties that induce perspiration to cool fever and stimulate the release of toxins from the body.

Diosgenin
An integral component in the synthesis of human sex hormones found in mexican yam (*Dioscorea* species) and fenugreek (*Trigonella foenum-graecum*).

Diuretic
An herb or medicine with properties that stimulate urination to relieve bloating and rid the body of excess water.

Digital Vaporization Technology
Advanced vaporization technique utilizing digital technology to maintain correct temperatures for each substance to avoid danger of combustion.

Dioxin
A heart medication derived from the from the common foxglove (*Digitalis purpurea*).

Emetic
An herb or medicine with properties that induce vomiting.

Emollient
An herb or medicine applied externally to soothe and protect the skin.

Enfleurage
Method that extracts the essential oils of plant matter through their absorption in oils of higher density and fat content.

Environmental Tobacco Smoke (ETS)
Also known as second-hand smoke. This includes both exhaled smoke and side-stream smoke from a burning cigarette, cigar, or pipe.

Essential Oil
A volatile oil, usually having the characteristic odor or flavor of the plant from which it is derived, released in vapor during the art of vaporization.

Expectorant
An herb or medicine that aids in the elimination of excess mucus in the respiratory system.

Expression
Method that uses pressure to extract the essential oils of a plant.

Heang
The Chinese word representing perfume, incense, and fragrance.

Hepatic
An herb or medicine with properties that fortify the liver and increase bile flow.

Hypnotic
A powerful sedative that induces a restorative sleep.

Hypotensive
An herb or medicine that regulates high blood pressure.

Holistic
A philosophy that emphasizes the importance of the whole and the interdependence of its parts. Holistic medicine believes the mind and the body should each be treated with direct regard to the other.

Ingestion
To take into the body by the mouth for digestion or absorption.

Kyphi
An ancient Egyptian aromatic blend used for incense and often offered to the sun-god, Ra.

Laxative (Aperient)
An herb or medicine that stimulates bowel movement.

Life Force
The vital energy that drives and enforces all life.

Limbic System
A group of related brain structures that play a significant role in emotion, motivation, and autonomic response.

Morphine
An analgesic and sedative derviced from the opium poppy (*Papaver rhoeas*).

Naturopathic
A system of therapy that relies on natural remedies to treat illness. Approaches include individual or combinations of remedies such as herbology, diet, exercise, and massage.

Nervine
An herb or medicine that regulates the nervous system through either a stimulating or relaxing effect.

NicoHale
An innovative smoking cessation product that utilizes the latest vaporization technology. Produced by Advanced Inhalation Revolutions, Inc.

Nostradamus
French physician, astrologer, and mystic who in 1555 wrote his infamous book of prophesy entitled *Centuries*.

Particulate Matter
Term to describe the combustion by-products, such as tar, found in tobacco smoke.

Pectoral
An herb or medicine that aids and strengthens the respiratory system.

Peptide
Two or more amino acids held together by peptide bonds.

Phytotechnician
One trained in the nature and elements of plant life and skilled in its application for human wellness.

Phyto-Vaporization
The principles of vaporization as applied to plant material.

Pranna
Ancient Indian term for "inner energy" and life force.

Pryolysis
The denaturization of matter by excessive heat.

Protein
Any of a large group of nitrogenous organic compounds that consist of long strings of amino acids and are essential constituents of living cells.

Quinine
An anti-malarial medication derived from various species of cinchona or Peruvian bark.

Solvent Extraction
A method of extracting the essential oils of plant matter through their absorption in alcohol.

Sedative
An herb or medicine with properties that reduce stress and soothe the nervous system.

Steam Distillation
A method that uses steam to extract the essential oils from plant matter.

Stimulant
An herb or medicine that increases energy and circulation and invigorates physiological functioning.

Tonic
An herb or medicine that stimulates overall health by increasing circulation and improving the absorption of vital nutrients to individual organs.

Tubocurarine
A powerful muscle derived from the plant curare (*Chondrondendron tomestosum*).

Unguent
A salve for soothing or healing; an ointment.

Vasodilator
An herb or medicine with properties that dilate blood vessels for increased circulation.

Volatilization
The degree to which a matter is easily vaporized or volatized.

Vulnerary
An herb or medicine, externally applied, that aids in the healing of wounds.

Yin and Yang
Chinese philosophy of two opposing principles that together give balance and harmony to the individual and the universe.

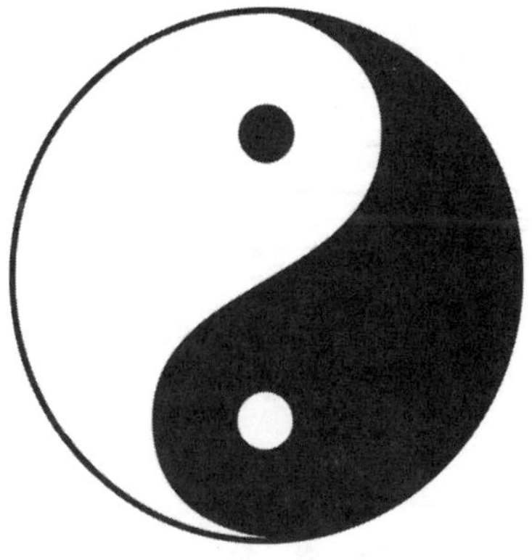

Herbal Index

A

B

C

D

E

F

G

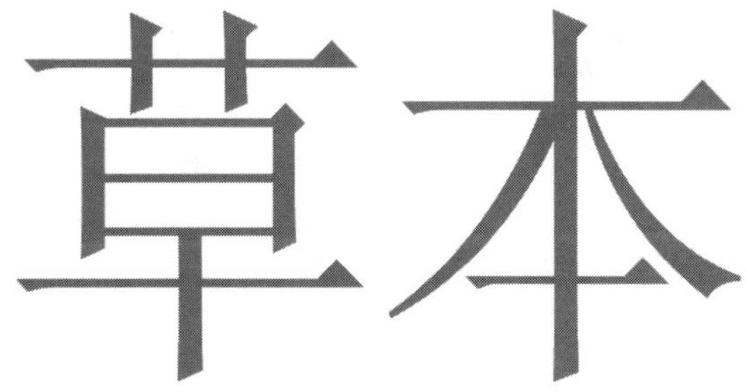
草本

About the Authors

SHAAHIN SEAN CHEYENE

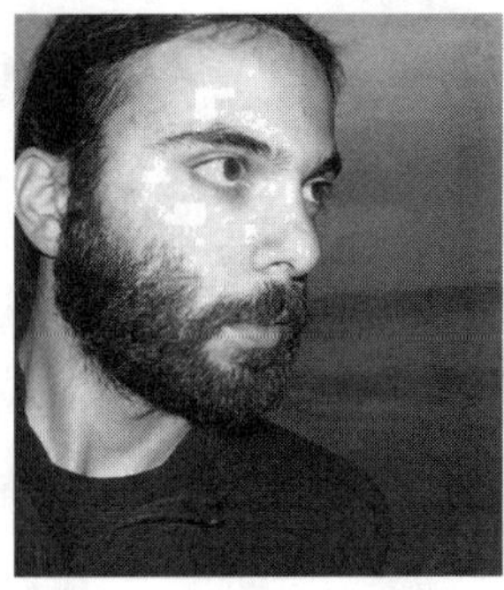
Photo by Asa Soltan Rahmati

Shaahin Sean Cheyene is a prominent herbalist and naturopath best known for his groundbreaking herbal formulations of the 1990s. He is a recognized authority on the development and marketing of smoking cessation technology, aromatherapy, herbal products and digital delivery technology. A member of the American Holistic Health Association, the United Nations Association, the American Civil Liberties Association (ACLU), and the American Botanical Council, Cheyene is a passionate supporter of complementary and alternative medicines.

Cheyene travels extensively to offer his consulting services to individuals and corporations across the globe, including those in the United States, Europe, Japan, Africa, South America, Central America, and Australia. Cheyene's expertise has benefited clients on nearly every continent.

Descended from several generations of naturopaths and herbalists from the countryside of Iran, Cheyene deeply believes in phytotechnology and the profound impact of digital vaporization on the future of human wellness.

JULIE ANN MARRA (RESEARCH ASSISTANT)

Julie Ann Marra is a professional writer with an enthusiasm for herbalism, nutrition, and holistic wellness. She is an avid supporter of vaporization technology and the freedom of choice in smoking cessation. She is a world traveler with an enveloping interest in varying cultures. Julie is a member of the National Writers Union, the International Women's Writing Guild and the Rittenhouse Writer's Group, with nationally published short fiction. She is currently researching a novel based on the changing roles of women in Indian society, and a collection of short stories entitled, *Wayward: Buses and Dust.*

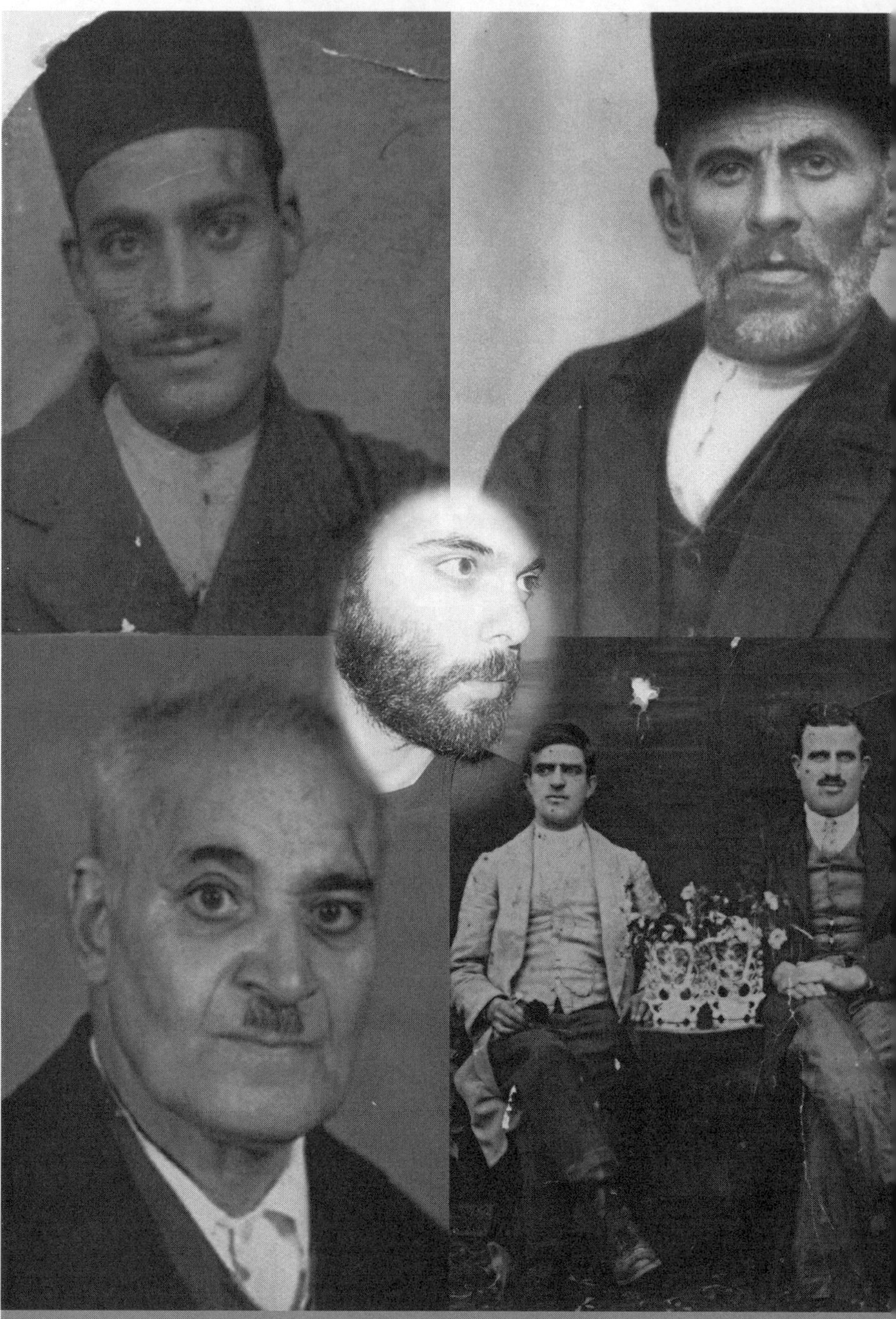

Cheyene is descended from several generations of naturopaths and herbalists from the countryside of Iran.